HEART HEALTHY COOKBOOK FOR BEGINNERS

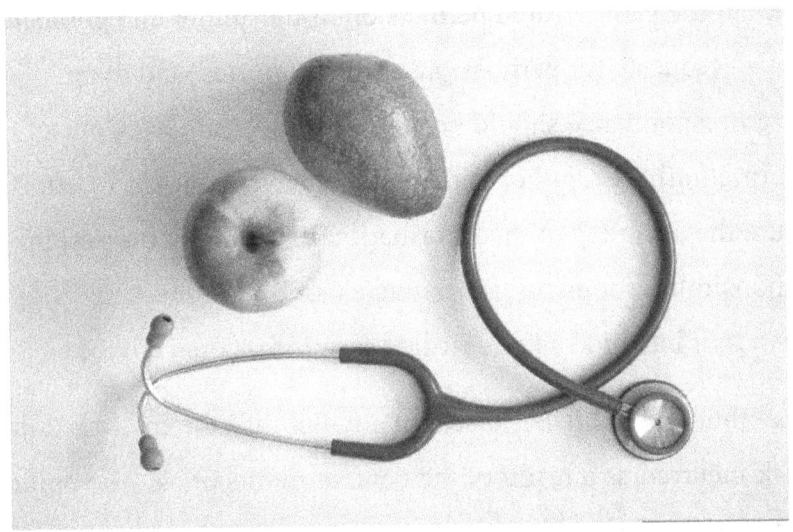

Quick, Easy and Tasty Low Sodium and Low- Fat Recipes with a 30 Days Meal Plan to Manage Your Body Weight, Blood Pressure and Cholesterol Level

Catherine Ellis

Copyright © 2023 by [Catherine Ellis]

All rights reserved. No part of this book may be reproduced, stored in a retrieval system, or transmitted in any form or by any means, electronic, mechanical, photocopying, recording, or otherwise, without the prior written permission of the author and publisher. Requests for permissions, press inquiries, and other correspondence should be addressed to [Author's Contact Information]. The author and publisher have made every effort to ensure the accuracy of the information in this book but assume no responsibility for errors, inaccuracies, or omissions. This book is not intended as a substitute for professional advice.

The author and publisher disclaim any liability for any loss, injury, or risk incurred as a result of the content in this book. The opinions expressed are those of the author and do not necessarily reflect the views of any organization or entity mentioned.

TABLE OF CONTENT

INTRODUCTION 5

  Understanding, Importance and Factors Affecting Heart Healthy 7

  The Importance of Heart Health 7

  Risk Factors 8

  Maintaining a Heart-Healthy Lifestyle: 8

  The Role of Medical Professionals 9

  Nutritional Guidelines for Heart Health 10

  Understanding Good and Bad Fats 13

CHAPTER 1 19

  Whole Grain Pasta Recipes 19

CHAPTER 2 33

  Poultry, Fish and Seafood Recipes 33

CHAPTER 3 45

  Salad Recipes 45

CHAPTER 4 59

Vegetable recipes 59

CHAPTER 5 73

Sauce and Stew Recipes 73

CHAPTER 6 85

Vegetarian Recipes 85

CHAPTER 7 103

Snacks and Desserts Recipes 103

Snacks: 103

Desserts: 106

CHAPTER 8 109

Smoothies Recipes 109

CHAPTER 9 117

30 Days Heart Healthy Meal Plan 117

CHAPTER 10 127

HEART HEALTHY FRUITS 127

CONCLUSION 131

INTRODUCTION

In the serene town of Willow brook, nestled among rolling hills and meandering streams, there lived a woman named Charlie. Once full of boundless energy and zest for life, Charlie found herself grappling with a health challenge that cast a shadow over her vibrant spirit heart issues.

Her heart troubles persisted despite multiple trips to the doctor and trials of different drugs. Frustration and a sense of helplessness settled in, prompting Charlie to seek alternative paths to wellness.

She had not yet looked into a solution until she came across a website late one night in the peaceful seclusion of her own house that enlighten on heart-healthy cookbook.

Intrigued and desperate for a solution, Charlie delved into the digital realm of nutritious recipes crafted explicitly for heart health. Authored by a renowned nutritionist, the cookbook unfolded a treasure trove of information on nutrient-rich ingredients and mindful cooking techniques.

Determined to take charge of her well-being, Charlie purchased the cookbook and embarked on a culinary journey that would soon transform her life.

The once-neglected kitchen now buzzed with activity as Charlie experimented with the diverse and tantalizing recipes.

As days turned into weeks, Charlie began to notice subtle but significant changes in her health. The nagging pain in her chest subsided, and she began to feel more alive every day. The heart healthy meals not only nourished her body but also became a source of joy and satisfaction.

One of the cookbook's most remarkable benefits for Charlie was the ability to enjoy a rich variety of flavors and textures without compromising on her health. The days of boring, restrictive diets were long gone, and she now enjoyed every meal as a celebration of flavor and health.

Word of Charlie's transformative journey spread throughout Willow brook, sparking curiosity and interest among her friends and neighbors.

Eager to share her newfound wisdom, Charlie became a beacon of inspiration, guiding others toward heart-healthy choices and mindful eating.

In the heart of the community, the local farmers' market flourished as demand for fresh, wholesome ingredients surged. Cooking became a communal experience, bringing people together to share not only delicious meals but also the joy of cultivating a healthier lifestyle.

As the sun dipped below the horizon, casting a warm glow over Willow brook, Charlie sat at her table, surrounded by the aroma of a heart-healthy dinner. Grateful for the cookbook that had not only solved her heart issues but had also ignited a positive change in her community, Charlie reveled in the newfound vitality that radiated from within.

Understanding, Importance and Factors Affecting Heart Healthy

Heart health is a crucial aspect of overall well-being, and a proactive approach to maintaining a healthy heart is essential for a long and fulfilling life.

Here's a comprehensive look at understanding heart health, including key factors, lifestyle choices, and strategies to promote cardiovascular well-being.

The Importance of Heart Health:

The heart is an essential organ that pumps blood throughout the body to carry nutrients and oxygen. Maintaining a healthy heart is fundamental to overall health and longevity.

Heart diseases, including coronary artery disease, heart failure, and arrhythmias, can significantly impact quality of life and pose serious health risks.

Risk Factors:

Unhealthy Diet: Diets high in saturated fats, trans fats, sodium, and cholesterol can contribute to heart disease.

Physical Inactivity: Lack of exercise is a significant risk factor for heart issues. The heart needs regular physical activity to stay healthy.

Smoking: Tobacco smoke contains chemicals that can damage blood vessels, leading to heart problems.

Excessive Alcohol Consumption: Drinking too much alcohol can elevate blood pressure and contribute to heart disease.

Genetics: Family history plays a role, as some heart conditions have a genetic component.

Maintaining a Heart-Healthy Lifestyle:

Balanced Diet: Emphasize fruits, vegetables, whole grains, lean proteins, and healthy fats. Restrict your consumption of processed meals, sweetened beverages, and too much salt.

Regular Exercise: Try to get in at least 150 minutes a week of moderate-to-intense physical activity.

This can include activities such as brisk walking, jogging, swimming, or cycling.

Smoking Cessation: Quitting smoking is one of the most significant steps towards improving heart health.

Moderate Alcohol Consumption: If you decide to have a drink, make sure it's small. For women, this usually translates to a maximum of one drink per day and a maximum of two drinks per day for men

Regular Check-Ups: Schedule regular health check-ups to monitor blood pressure, cholesterol levels, and other key indicators of heart health.

Stress Management: Chronic stress can contribute to heart problems. Adopt stress-reducing techniques such as meditation, yoga, or deep breathing exercises.

The Role of Medical Professionals:

Maintaining and monitoring heart health requires routine visits with medical specialists, such as cardiologists and primary care physicians

Diagnostic tests such as blood pressure measurements, cholesterol screenings, and electrocardiograms (ECGs) help assess cardiovascular risk and identify potential issues.

Heart-Healthy Resources:

Utilize reputable sources for heart-healthy recipes, exercise routines, and lifestyle tips.

Think about the educational resources offered by respectable medical facilities and heart health organizations

Understanding heart health involves a holistic approach encompassing lifestyle choices, risk factor management, and regular medical assessments.

By adopting heart-healthy habits and staying informed, individuals can take proactive steps to promote cardiovascular well-being and enjoy a healthier, more fulfilling life.

Nutritional Guidelines for Heart Health

Maintaining a heart-healthy diet is integral to overall cardiovascular well-being. Adopting proper nutritional habits can significantly reduce the risk of heart disease and contribute to a healthier, more robust life.

Here's a concise exploration of nutritional guidelines for heart health:

Emphasize Fruits and Vegetables:

Colorful fruits and vegetables are rich in vitamins, minerals, and antioxidants that support heart health.

Aim to include a variety of fruits and vegetables in different colors to ensure a diverse range of nutrients.

Choose Whole Grains:

For whole grains like whole wheat, quinoa, brown rice, and oats, optional. These grains provide fiber, which aids in maintaining healthy cholesterol levels and promotes heart health.

Prioritize Lean Proteins:

Include lean protein sources like poultry, fish, legumes, and tofu. These proteins are lower in saturated fats, reducing the risk of cholesterol-related heart issues.

Healthy Fats:

Include foods like avocados, almonds, seeds, and olive oil that are good sources of fat. These fats can positively impact cholesterol levels and overall heart health.

Limit Saturated and Trans Fats:

Reduce the intake of saturated and trans fats found in processed foods, fried items, and certain baked goods. These fats raise the risk of heart disease and can contribute to high cholesterol levels.

Control Portion Sizes:

Be mindful of portion sizes to prevent overeating. Be mindful of your body's signals of hunger and fullness, and refrain from consuming excessive amounts of high-calorie, low-nutrient foods.

Manage Sodium Intake:

Foods heavy in sodium should be consumed in moderation since too much salt can raise blood pressure. Optional for herbs and spices for flavoring instead of relying on salt.

Moderate Sugar Intake:

Minimize the intake of added sugars found in sugary beverages, candies, and processed snacks. High sugar consumption is linked to obesity and an increased risk of heart disease.

Stay Hydrated:

Maintain adequate hydration by drinking water throughout the day. Water promotes general health and facilitates a more effective heartbeat.

Limit Alcohol Consumption:

If you decide to consume alcohol, do so sparingly. This translates to one drink for women and two for men per day for the majority of adults

Consider Dietary Supplements:

Consult with a healthcare professional about the need for supplements, such as omega-3 fatty acids or specific vitamins, to complement a heart-healthy diet.

Customize to Individual Needs:

Recognize that individual nutritional needs may vary. Factors such as age, gender, activity level, and existing health conditions should be considered when tailoring a heart-healthy diet.

Eating a heart-healthy diet requires making thoughtful, balanced dietary selections. By incorporating nutrient-rich foods, minimizing unhealthy fats and sugars, and maintaining overall dietary balance, individuals can promote heart health and reduce the risk of cardiovascular diseases.

Always consult with a healthcare professional or a registered dietitian for personalized advice based on individual health needs and goals.

Understanding Good and Bad Fats

Monounsaturated Fats: Found in olive oil, avocados, nuts, and seeds, monounsaturated fats can help lower bad cholesterol levels (LDL) and reduce the risk of heart disease.

Fats play a crucial role in the functioning of our bodies, but not all fats are created equal. Distinguishing between good and bad fats is essential for maintaining heart health and preventing cardiovascular issues. Here's a brief and comprehensive guide to understanding the impact of fats on heart health:

Good Fats - Unsaturated Fats:

Polyunsaturated Fats: Sources include fatty fish (salmon, mackerel), flaxseeds, walnuts, and vegetable oils. These fats contain omega-3 and omega-6 fatty acids, which contribute to heart health by reducing inflammation and supporting overall cardiovascular function.

Bad Fats - Saturated Fats:

Commonly found in red meat, full-fat dairy products, butter, and tropical oils (coconut oil, palm oil), saturated fats can raise LDL cholesterol levels, increasing the risk of heart disease.

Limiting the intake of saturated fats is crucial for maintaining a heart-healthy diet.

Trans Fats:

Trans fats are artificially created fats through a process called hydrogenation, often used in processed and packaged foods to extend shelf life.

Trans fats significantly raise LDL cholesterol while lowering HDL cholesterol (good cholesterol), making them particularly detrimental to heart health.

Many health authorities recommend avoiding trans fats altogether.

Understanding Cholesterol:

Cholesterol is a fatty substance that is crucial for building cells and producing hormones. However, too much LDL cholesterol can build up in arteries, leading to atherosclerosis and an increased risk of heart disease.

Conversely, HDL cholesterol lowers the risk of heart problems by assisting in the removal of LDL cholesterol from the bloodstream

Balancing Fats in the Diet:

A heart-healthy diet emphasizes replacing saturated and trans fats with unsaturated fats.

Choose lean protein sources, incorporate fatty fish, and use plant-based oils such as olive oil or canola oil for cooking.

Nuts, seeds, and avocados are excellent snacks that provide healthy fats and additional nutrients.

Reading Nutrition Labels:

When grocery shopping, pay attention to food labels. Check for the presence of saturated and trans fats in processed foods.

Optional for products with lower saturated and trans-fat content and higher amounts of unsaturated fats.

Cooking Methods Matter:

Instead of frying, choose healthy cooking techniques like baking, grilling, steaming, or sautéing

Trim visible fats from meat and remove the skin from poultry to reduce saturated fat intake.

Consulting with Healthcare Professionals:

Individuals with specific health concerns or conditions should consult with healthcare professionals or registered dietitians to create a personalized dietary plan.

Understanding good and bad fats is a key component of promoting heart health. By incorporating unsaturated fats while limiting saturated and trans fats, individuals can make informed dietary choices that contribute to overall cardiovascular well-being. A balanced and mindful approach to fat intake, combined with a healthy lifestyle, is integral to reducing the risk of heart disease.

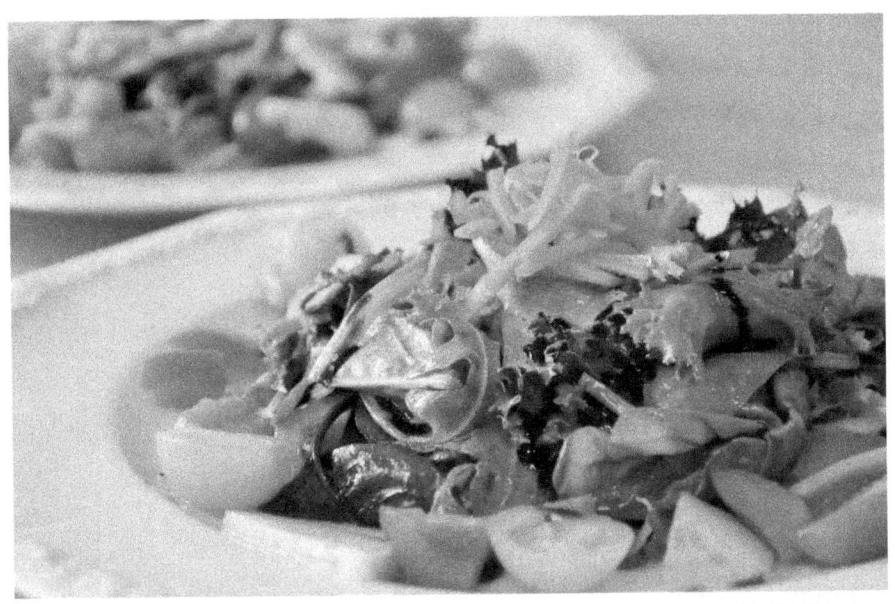
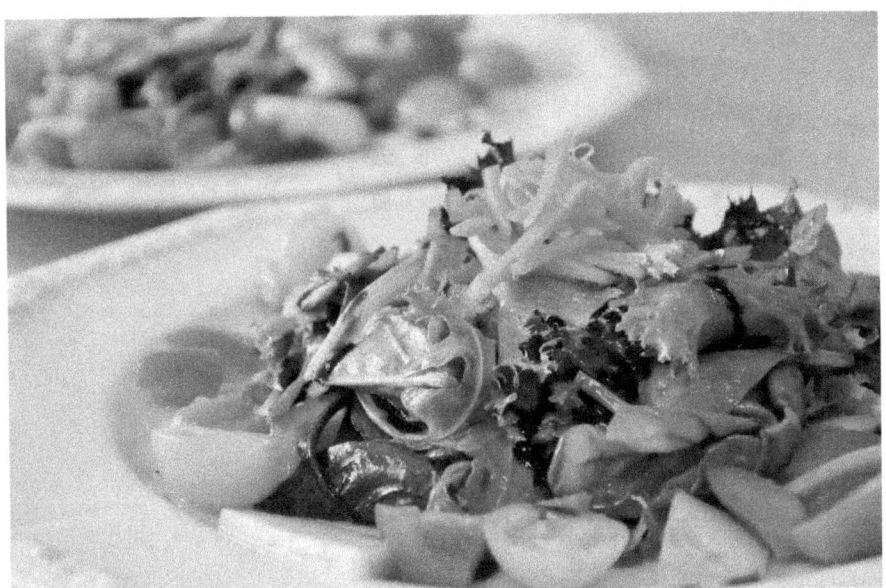

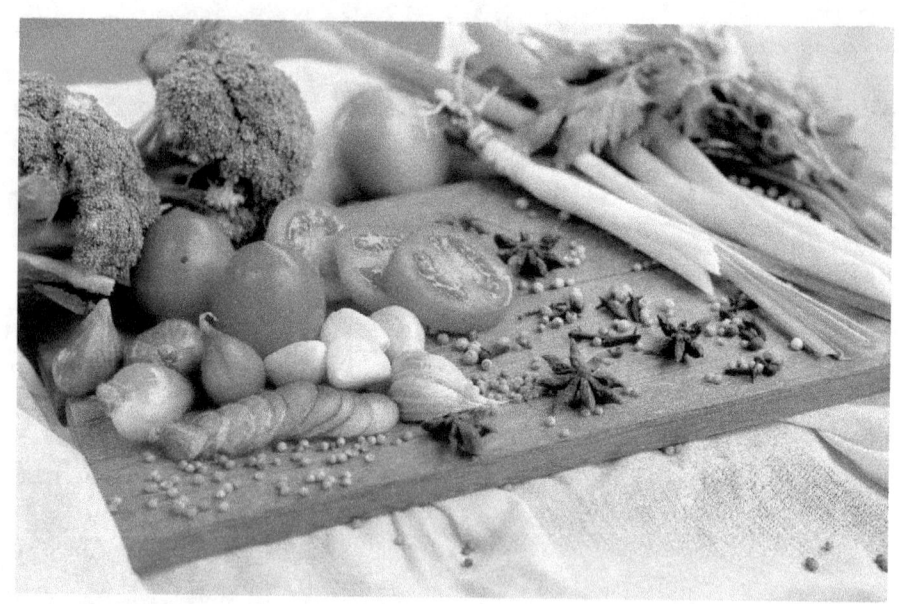

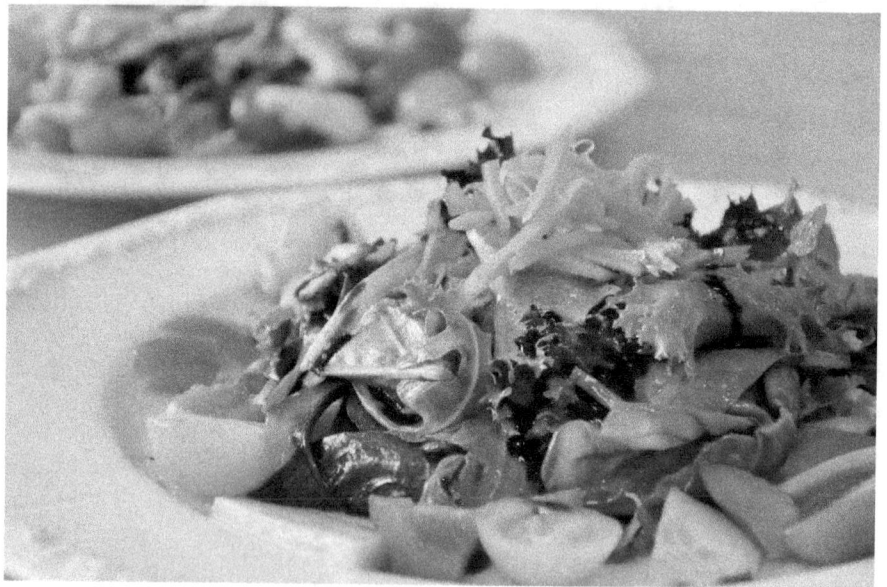

CHAPTER 1

Whole Grain Pasta Recipes

1. Mediterranean Whole Grain Pasta Salad

Introduction: This refreshing pasta salad is packed with heart-healthy ingredients inspired by the Mediterranean diet.

Ingredients:

2 cups whole grain penne pasta

1 cup cherry tomatoes, halved

1 cucumber, diced

1/2 cup Kalamata olives, sliced

1/4 cup feta cheese, crumbled

1/4 cup extra-virgin olive oil

2 tablespoons balsamic vinegar

1 teaspoon dried oregano

Salt and pepper to taste

Instructions:

Pasta should be cooked as directed on the package, drained, and then allowed to cool

In a large bowl, combine pasta, tomatoes, cucumber, olives, and feta.

Mix the olive oil, balsamic vinegar, oregano, salt, and pepper in a small basin.

After adding the dressing to the spaghetti mixture, gently toss to blend.

Let it cool for a minimum of half an hour before serving

Prep Time: 15 minutes

2. Spinach and Garlic Whole Grain Spaghetti

Introduction: This garlic-infused whole grain spaghetti is paired with nutrient-rich spinach for a simple and heart-healthy dish.

Ingredients:

8 oz whole grain spaghetti

2 tablespoons olive oil

4 cloves garlic, minced

4 cups fresh spinach

1/4 teaspoon red pepper flakes (optional)

Salt and black pepper to taste

Grated Parmesan cheese for garnish

Instructions:

After cooking spaghetti as directed on the package, drain and set aside.

Heat the olive oil in a big skillet over medium heat. When aromatic, add the minced garlic and sauté it

Add spinach to the skillet and cook until wilted. Black pepper, salt, and red pepper flakes are used for seasoning.

Toss the cooked spaghetti into the skillet and mix until well combined.

Serve hot, garnished with grated Parmesan cheese.

Prep Time: 20 minutes

3. Tomato and Basil Whole Wheat Fusilli

Introduction: This classic combination of tomatoes and basil creates a flavorful and heart-healthy whole wheat fusilli dish.

Ingredients:

2 cups whole wheat fusilli pasta

1 tablespoon olive oil

3 cloves garlic, minced

2 cups cherry tomatoes, halved

1/2 cup fresh basil, chopped

1/4 cup grated Pecorino Romano cheese

Salt and black pepper to taste

Instructions:

Cook fusilli according to package instructions, drain, and set aside.

Warm up the olive oil in a big skillet over medium heat. Add minced garlic and sauté until golden.

Add cherry tomatoes to the pan and cook until they release their juices.

Toss in the cooked fusilli and fresh basil. Stir until well combined.

Season with salt and black pepper, and sprinkle Pecorino Romano cheese on top before serving.

Prep Time: 25 minutes

4. Lemon Garlic Shrimp and Whole Grain Linguine

Introduction: This light and zesty dish combine whole grain linguine with succulent shrimp, making it a heart-healthy delight.

Ingredients:

8 oz whole grain linguine

1 lb shrimp, peeled and deveined

3 tablespoons olive oil

4 cloves garlic, minced

Zest and juice of 1 lemon

1/4 cup fresh parsley, chopped

Salt and black pepper to taste

Instructions:

Cook linguine according to package instructions, drain, and set aside.

Heat the olive oil in a big skillet over medium heat. When aromatic, add the minced garlic and sauté it.

When the shrimp are pink and opaque, add them to the skillet and simmer

Toss the cooked linguine into the skillet. Add the fresh parsley, lemon juice, and zest. Mix well.

Before serving, add a dash of black pepper and salt.

Prep Time: 30 minutes

5. Vegetarian Whole Grain Orzo Primavera

Introduction: Loaded with colorful vegetables, this whole grain orzo primavera is a hearty and heart-healthy choice for vegetarians.

Ingredients:

1 cup whole grain orzo pasta

2 tablespoons olive oil

1 onion, diced

2 carrots, julienned

1 bell pepper (any color), sliced

1 zucchini, diced

1 cup cherry tomatoes, halved

1/2 cup frozen peas

1/4 cup fresh basil, chopped

1/4 cup grated Parmesan cheese

Salt and black pepper to taste

Instructions:

Prepare the orzo as directed on the package, pour out the excess, and reserve.

Warm up the olive oil in a big skillet over medium heat. Add onion slices and cook until transparent.

Add carrots, bell pepper, zucchini, cherry tomatoes, and peas. Cook until vegetables are tender.

Toss the cooked orzo into the pan, add fresh basil, and mix well.

Season with salt and black pepper, and sprinkle Parmesan cheese on top before serving.

Prep Time: 25 minutes

6. Chicken and Broccoli Whole Wheat Penne Alfredo

Introduction: A protein-packed dish featuring whole wheat penne, chicken, and broccoli in a creamy Alfredo sauce for a satisfying and heart-healthy meal.

Ingredients:

2 cups whole wheat penne pasta

1 lb boneless, skinless chicken breast, diced

2 tablespoons olive oil

2 cups broccoli florets

2 cloves garlic, minced

1 cup low-fat milk

1 cup grated Parmesan cheese

Salt and black pepper to taste

Instructions:

Cook penne according to package instructions, drain, and set aside.

Olive oil should be heated over medium heat in a big skillet. Add diced chicken and cook until browned.

Add broccoli and minced garlic to the skillet. Cook until broccoli is tender.

Pour in the milk and Parmesan cheese, stirring until the cheese is melted and the sauce is creamy.

Coat the cooked penne with the Alfredo sauce by tossing it into the skillet. Before serving, add a dash of black pepper and salt

Prep Time: 35 minutes

7. Roasted Red Pepper and Artichoke Whole Grain Farfalle

Introduction: This vibrant dish features whole grain farfalle pasta with the rich flavors of roasted red pepper and artichoke.

Ingredients:

2 cups whole grain farfalle pasta

One 12-oz container of chopped, drained, and roasted red peppers

One 14-oz can of drained and quartered artichoke hearts

1/4 cup pine nuts, toasted

2 tablespoons olive oil

2 cloves garlic, minced

Instruction

Follow the directions on the package to cook the farfalle, then drain and set aside.

Warm up the olive oil in a big skillet over medium heat. Add the minced garlic and cook it until fragrant

Add the chopped roasted red peppers and quartered artichoke hearts to the pan. Cook until heated through.

Toss the cooked farfalle into the pan, ensuring it's well-coated with the flavorful mixture.

Sprinkle toasted pine nuts over the pasta for added crunch and depth of flavor.

Season with salt and black pepper to taste. Serve warm.

Prep Time: 25 minutes

8. Whole Grain Penne with Tomato and Chickpea Sauce

Introduction: This protein-rich pasta dish combines whole grain penne with a hearty tomato and chickpea sauce, providing a satisfying and heart-healthy option.

Ingredients:

2 cups whole grain penne pasta

One can (15 oz) of rinsed and drained chickpeas

1 can (28 oz) crushed tomatoes

1 onion, finely chopped

3 cloves garlic, minced

2 tablespoons olive oil

1 teaspoon dried oregano

1/2 teaspoon red pepper flakes (optional)

Salt and black pepper to taste

Fresh parsley for garnish

Instructions:

Cook penne according to package instructions, drain, and set aside.

Olive oil should be heated over medium heat in a big saucepan. When the onion is soft, add it diced and sauté it

Add minced garlic and cook until fragrant. Stir in crushed tomatoes, chickpeas, oregano, and red pepper flakes.

Allow the flavors to mingle by simmering the sauce for 15 to 20 minutes

Toss the cooked penne into the sauce, ensuring it's well-coated. Season with salt and black pepper.

Garnish with fresh parsley before serving.

Prep Time: 30 minutes

9. Spaghetti with Turkey and Mushroom Bolognese

Introduction: This lean turkey and mushroom Bolognese over whole wheat spaghetti offers a heart-healthy twist on a classic comfort dish.

Ingredients:

8 oz whole wheat spaghetti

1 lb lean ground turkey

2 cups cremini mushrooms, finely chopped

1 onion, diced

3 cloves garlic, minced

1 can (28 oz) crushed tomatoes

2 tablespoons tomato paste

1 teaspoon dried thyme

Salt and black pepper to taste

Fresh basil for garnish

Instructions:

After cooking spaghetti as directed on the package, drain and set aside

In a large skillet, brown the ground turkey over medium heat. Add chopped mushrooms, onion, and garlic.

Stir in crushed tomatoes, tomato paste, and dried thyme. Simmer for 15-20 minutes.

Season the Bolognese sauce with salt and black pepper to taste.

Toss the cooked spaghetti into the sauce until well-coated. Garnish with fresh basil before serving.

Prep Time: 35 minutes

10. Pesto-topped whole-grain rotini with cherry tomatoes

Introduction: This quick and flavorful dish combines whole grain rotini with a vibrant pesto sauce and juicy cherry tomatoes for a heart-healthy delight.

Ingredients:

2 cups whole grain rotini pasta

1 cup cherry tomatoes, halved

1/2 cup pine nuts, toasted

1 cup fresh basil leaves

1/2 cup grated Parmesan cheese

2 cloves garlic

1/2 cup extra-virgin olive oil

Salt and black pepper to taste

Instructions:

Cook the rotini as directed on the box, then drain and set aside

In a food processor, combine basil, garlic, pine nuts, and Parmesan cheese. Pulse until finely chopped.

With the processor running, slowly add the olive oil until a smooth pesto sauce form

Toss the cooked rotini with the pesto sauce, ensuring even coating.

Gently fold in the halved cherry tomatoes. Season with salt and black pepper.

If preferred, top warm servings with more Parmesan cheese.

Prep Time: 20 minutes

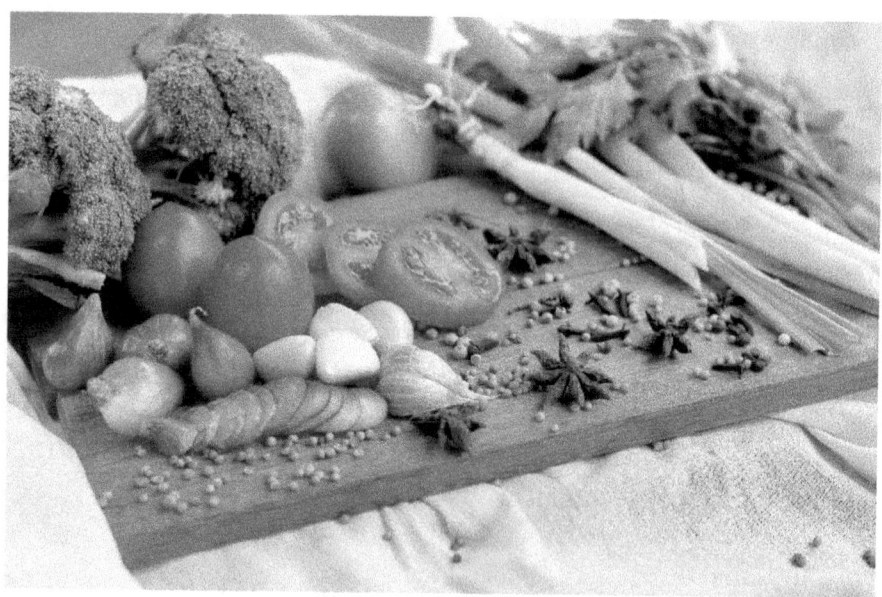

CHAPTER 2

Poultry, Fish and Seafood Recipes

1. Grilled Lemon Herb Chicken Breast

Introduction:

This simple and flavorful grilled chicken recipe is low in saturated fats and high in lean protein, making it a heart-healthy option.

Ingredients:

4 boneless, skinless chicken breasts

2 tablespoons olive oil

1 lemon (juiced)

2 cloves garlic (minced)

1 teaspoon dried oregano

Salt and pepper to taste

Instructions:

Combine the olive oil, lemon juice, dried oregano, minced garlic, salt, and pepper in a bowl.

For a minimum of half an hour, marinate chicken breasts in the marinade

Preheat grill to medium-high heat.

Grill chicken for 6-8 minutes per side or until cooked through.

Prep Time: 40 minutes

2. Baked Salmon with Dill Sauce

Introduction:

Omega-3 fatty acids, which are abundant in salmon, are good for the heart. This baked salmon with dill sauce is a tasty and nutritious choice.

Ingredients:

4 salmon fillets

2 tablespoons olive oil

1 lemon (sliced)

2 tablespoons fresh dill (chopped)

Salt and pepper to taste

Instructions:

Preheat oven to 375°F (190°C).

Place salmon fillets on a baking sheet.

Drizzle with olive oil, sprinkle with salt, pepper, and fresh dill.

Top each fillet with lemon slices.

Bake for 15 to 20 minutes, or until a fork can easily pierce the salmon

Prep Time: 25 minutes

3. Shrimp and Quinoa Salad

Introduction:

Packed with protein and fiber, this shrimp and quinoa salad is light, refreshing, and perfect for a heart-healthy lunch.

Ingredients:

1 cup quinoa (cooked)

1 pound shrimp (peeled and deveined)

1 cup cherry tomatoes (halved)

1 cucumber (diced)

1/4 cup red onion (finely chopped)

2 tablespoons fresh parsley (chopped)

2 tablespoons olive oil

1 lemon (juiced)

Salt and pepper to taste

Instructions:

Quinoa, shrimp, tomatoes, cucumber, red onion, and parsley should all be combined in a big bowl.

Mix the olive oil, lemon juice, salt, and pepper in a small bowl.

After adding the dressing to the salad, toss to mix

Prep Time: 30 minutes

4. Grilled Tuna Steaks with Mango Salsa

Introduction:

Tuna is a great source of omega-3 fatty acids. This grilled tuna with mango salsa is a delicious way to incorporate heart-healthy nutrients.

Ingredients:

4 tuna steaks

1 tablespoon olive oil

1 teaspoon ground cumin

Salt and pepper to taste

Mango Salsa:

1 ripe mango (diced)

1/2 red onion (finely chopped)

1 jalapeño (seeded and diced)

2 tablespoons fresh cilantro (chopped)

1 lime (juiced)

Instructions:

Rub tuna steaks with olive oil, cumin, salt, and pepper.

Grill tuna for 2-3 minutes per side.

In a bowl, mix mango, red onion, jalapeño, cilantro, and lime juice for salsa.

Serve tuna steaks with mango salsa on top.

Prep Time: 25 minutes

5. Lemon Garlic Herb Roasted Chicken Thighs

Introduction:

These roasted chicken thighs are juicy and flavorful, with heart-healthy olive oil and a burst of citrusy freshness from lemon.

Ingredients:

8 chicken thighs (bone-in, skin-on)

3 tablespoons olive oil

3 cloves garlic (minced)

1 lemon (zested and juiced)

1 teaspoon dried thyme

Salt and pepper to taste

Instructions:

Preheat oven to 400°F (200°C).

In a bowl, mix olive oil, minced garlic, lemon zest, lemon juice, thyme, salt, and pepper.

Rub the mixture over chicken thighs.

Roast in the oven for 35-40 minutes or until the internal temperature reaches 165°F (74°C).

Prep Time: 50 minutes

6. Broiled Lemon Garlic Shrimp Skewers

Introduction:

These broiled shrimp skewers are quick to make and bursting with lemon and garlic flavor, providing a heart-healthy dose of protein.

Ingredients:

1 pound large shrimp (peeled and deveined)

2 tablespoons olive oil

3 cloves garlic (minced)

1 lemon (zested and juiced)

1 teaspoon paprika

Salt and pepper to taste

Instructions:

Preheat the broiler.

Olive oil, minced garlic, lemon zest, lemon juice, paprika, salt, and pepper should all be combined in a bowl

Thread shrimp onto skewers and brush with the lemon-garlic mixture.

Bake the shrimp for 3–4 minutes on each side, or until they are opaque

Prep Time: 20 minutes

7. Mediterranean Baked Cod

Introduction:

This Mediterranean-inspired baked cod is rich in heart-healthy omega-3 fatty acids and features a delightful blend of herbs and vegetables.

Ingredients:

4 cod fillets

2 tablespoons olive oil

1 teaspoon dried oregano

1 teaspoon dried thyme

1 cup cherry tomatoes (halved)

1/2 cup Kalamata olives (pitted and sliced)

1/4 cup feta cheese (crumbled)

Instructions:

Preheat oven to 400°F (200°C).

Place cod fillets in a baking dish.

Drizzle with olive oil, sprinkle with oregano and thyme.

Add cherry tomatoes and Kalamata olives around the fish.

Fish should flake readily after 20 to 25 minutes in the oven.

Before serving, scatter the feta cheese on top

Prep Time: 30 minutes

8. Lemon Rosemary Roast Turkey Breast

Introduction:

This lean turkey breast is roasted with heart-healthy olive oil, lemon, and rosemary, creating a flavorful and satisfying dish.

Ingredients:

1 turkey breast (bone-in, skin-on)

3 tablespoons olive oil

2 lemons (zested and juiced)

2 tablespoons fresh rosemary (chopped)

Salt and pepper to taste

Instructions:

Preheat oven to 325°F (163°C).

In a bowl, mix olive oil, lemon zest, lemon juice, chopped rosemary, salt, and pepper.

Rub the mixture over the turkey breast.

Roast in the oven for 1.5 to 2 hours or until the internal temperature reaches 165°F (74°C).

Prep Time: 2 hours and 15 minutes

9. Garlic Butter Baked Salmon

Introduction:

This garlic butter baked salmon is not only delicious but also heart-healthy, thanks to the omega-3 fatty acids in salmon and the use of olive oil.

Ingredients:

4 salmon fillets

4 tablespoons unsalted butter (melted)

4 cloves garlic (minced)

2 tablespoons fresh parsley (chopped)

Salt and pepper to taste

Lemon wedges for serving

Instructions:

Preheat oven to 375°F (190°C).

Place salmon fillets on a baking sheet.

Melted butter, minced garlic, chopped parsley, salt, and pepper should all be combined in a small bowl

Brush the butter mixture over the salmon.

Bake the salmon for 15 to 20 minutes, or until it flake easily with a fork

Serve with lemon wedges.

Prep Time: 25 minutes

10. Lemon Garlic Grilled Swordfish

Introduction:

Swordfish is a hearty and meaty fish that pairs well with the bright flavors of lemon and garlic. This grilled swordfish is a delicious and heart-healthy option.

Ingredients:

4 swordfish steaks

3 tablespoons olive oil

2 cloves garlic (minced)

1 lemon (zested and juiced)

1 teaspoon dried oregano

Salt and pepper to taste

Instructions:

Preheat grill to medium-high heat.

In a bowl, mix olive oil, minced garlic, lemon zest, lemon juice, dried oregano, salt, and pepper.

Apply the lemon-garlic mixture on the swordfish steaks.

Grill for 4-5 minutes per side or until the fish is cooked through.

Prep Time: 30 minutes

CHAPTER 3

Salad Recipes

1. Mediterranean Quinoa Salad

Introduction: Embrace the flavors of the Mediterranean with this nutrient-packed quinoa salad.

Ingredients:

1 cup quinoa, cooked and cooled

1 cup cherry tomatoes, halved

1 cucumber, diced

1/2 cup Kalamata olives, pitted and sliced

1/4 cup red onion, finely chopped

1/2 cup feta cheese, crumbled

2 tablespoons extra-virgin olive oil

1 tablespoon red wine vinegar

Salt and pepper to taste

Instructions:

In a large bowl, combine quinoa, cherry tomatoes, cucumber, olives, red onion, and feta cheese.

Mix the olive oil, red wine vinegar, salt, and pepper in a small bowl.

After adding the dressing to the salad, gently toss to mix.

Let it cool for a minimum of half an hour before serving

Prep Time: 20 minutes

2. Kale and Berry Salad

Introduction: This vibrant salad is a powerhouse of antioxidants and heart-healthy nutrients.

Ingredients:

4 cups of chopped and massaged kale leaves

1 cup mixed berries (strawberries, blueberries, raspberries)

1/4 cup walnuts, chopped

1/4 cup feta cheese, crumbled

2 tablespoons balsamic vinaigrette dressing

1 tablespoon honey

Instructions:

In a large bowl, combine kale, mixed berries, walnuts, and feta cheese.

Drizzle balsamic vinaigrette and honey over the salad.

Toss well to coat the ingredients evenly.

Allow the salad to sit for 10 minutes before serving.

Prep Time: 15 minutes

3. Grilled Chicken Caesar Salad

Introduction: A heart-healthy twist on the classic Caesar salad with the addition of grilled chicken.

Ingredients:

2 boneless, skinless chicken breasts

1 head romaine lettuce, chopped

1/4 cup Parmesan cheese, grated

1/2 cup whole wheat croutons

2 tablespoons olive oil

1 clove garlic, minced

2 tablespoons Greek yogurt

1 tablespoon lemon juice

Salt and pepper to taste

Instructions:

Season chicken breasts with salt and pepper and grill until fully cooked.

Romaine lettuce, Parmesan cheese, and croutons should all be combined in a big bowl

In a small bowl, whisk together olive oil, garlic, Greek yogurt, lemon juice, salt, and pepper to create the dressing.

Slice the grilled chicken and place it on top of the salad.

Before serving, gently toss the salad with the dressing after pouring it over it

Prep Time: 25 minutes

4. Spinach and Quinoa Salad with Salmon

Introduction: A protein-packed salad featuring heart-healthy salmon and nutrient-rich spinach.

Ingredients:

2 cups baby spinach

1 cup quinoa, cooked and cooled

1/2 cup cherry tomatoes, halved

1/4 cup red bell pepper, diced

1/4 cup feta cheese, crumbled

1 grilled salmon fillet, flaked

2 tablespoons olive oil

1 tablespoon lemon juice

1 teaspoon Dijon mustard

Salt and pepper to taste

Instructions:

In a large bowl, combine baby spinach, quinoa, cherry tomatoes, red bell pepper, feta cheese, and flaked salmon.

Mix the olive oil, lemon juice, Dijon mustard, salt, and pepper in a small bowl.

Over the salad, drizzle with the dressing and toss lightly to mix

Serve immediately.

Prep Time: 30 minutes

5. Chickpea and Vegetable Salad

Introduction: Packed with fiber and protein, this chickpea salad is a heart-healthy delight.

Ingredients:

One can (15 oz) of rinsed and drained chickpeas

1 cup cherry tomatoes, halved

1 cucumber, diced

1/4 cup red onion, finely chopped

1/4 cup feta cheese, crumbled

2 tablespoons fresh parsley, chopped

3 tablespoons olive oil

2 tablespoons balsamic vinegar

Salt and pepper to taste

Instructions:

In a large bowl, combine chickpeas, cherry tomatoes, cucumber, red onion, feta cheese, and fresh parsley.

In a small bowl, whisk together olive oil, balsamic vinegar, salt, and pepper.

After adding the dressing to the salad, gently toss to mix.

Allow the salad to marinate in the refrigerator for at least 20 minutes before serving.

Prep Time: 15 minutes

6. Asian-Inspired Edamame Salad

Introduction: A colorful and protein-packed salad with the goodness of edamame and a zesty Asian-inspired dressing.

Ingredients:

2 cups shelled edamame, cooked and cooled

1 cup red cabbage, thinly sliced

1 carrot, julienned

1 red bell pepper, thinly sliced

1/4 cup green onions, chopped

1/4 cup cilantro, chopped

2 tablespoons sesame oil

1 tablespoon soy sauce

1 tablespoon rice vinegar

1 tablespoon honey

1 teaspoon fresh ginger, grated

Instructions:

In a large bowl, combine edamame, red cabbage, carrot, red bell pepper, green onions, and cilantro.

In a small bowl, whisk together sesame oil, soy sauce, rice vinegar, honey, and ginger to create the dressing.

Drizzle the salad with the dressing and thoroughly mix to coat

Allow the flavors to meld by refrigerating for at least 15 minutes before serving.

Prep Time: 20 minutes

7. Roasted Vegetable Quinoa Salad

Introduction: A satisfying and heart-healthy salad featuring roasted vegetables and protein-packed quinoa.

Ingredients:

1 cup quinoa, cooked and cooled

1 cup cherry tomatoes, halved

1 zucchini, diced

1 red bell pepper, diced

1 yellow bell pepper, diced

1 cup broccoli florets

2 tablespoons olive oil

1 teaspoon Italian seasoning

Salt and pepper to taste

2 tablespoons balsamic glaze

Instructions:

Preheat the oven to 400°F (200°C).

In a large baking pan, toss zucchini, red bell pepper, yellow bell pepper, and broccoli with olive oil, Italian seasoning, salt, and pepper.

Roast the vegetables for 20-25 minutes or until they are tender and slightly caramelized.

In a large bowl, combine quinoa, roasted vegetables, and cherry tomatoes.

Drizzle balsamic glaze over the salad and toss gently before serving.

Prep Time: 30 minutes

8. Tuna and White Bean Salad

Introduction: A protein-packed salad with the heart-healthy benefits of tuna and white beans.

Ingredients:

One can (5 oz) of drained tuna in water

One can (15 oz) of rinsed and drained white beans

1 cup cherry tomatoes, halved

1/4 cup red onion, finely chopped

2 tablespoons capers

2 tablespoons fresh parsley, chopped

2 tablespoons olive oil

1 tablespoon red wine vinegar

Salt and pepper to taste

Instructions:

In a large bowl, combine tuna, white beans, cherry tomatoes, red onion, capers, and fresh parsley.

Mix the olive oil, red wine vinegar, salt, and pepper in a small bowl.

After adding the dressing to the salad, gently toss to mix

Allow the salad to chill in the refrigerator for at least 15 minutes before serving.

Prep Time: 15 minutes

9. Strawberry Avocado Spinach Salad

Introduction: A refreshing and heart-healthy salad that combines the sweetness of strawberries with the creaminess of avocado.

Ingredients:

4 cups baby spinach

1 cup strawberries, sliced

1 avocado, diced

1/4 cup red onion, thinly sliced

1/4 cup feta cheese, crumbled

2 tablespoons balsamic vinaigrette dressing

1 tablespoon honey

2 tablespoons chopped almonds (optional)

Instructions:

In a large bowl, combine baby spinach, strawberries, avocado, red onion, and feta cheese.

Drizzle balsamic vinaigrette and honey over the salad.

Toss gently to coat the ingredients evenly.

If preferred, sprinkle chopped almonds on top, then serve right away

Prep Time: 15 minutes

10. Salmon and Avocado Caesar Salad

Introduction: A heart-healthy twist on the classic Caesar salad, featuring omega-3-rich salmon and creamy avocado.

Ingredients:

2 cups romaine lettuce, chopped

1/2 cup cherry tomatoes, halved

1/4 cup croutons

1/4 cup Parmesan cheese, grated

1/2 avocado, sliced

1 grilled salmon fillet, flaked

2 tablespoons Greek yogurt

1 tablespoon lemon juice

1 tablespoon olive oil

Salt and pepper to taste

Instructions:

In a large bowl, combine romaine lettuce, cherry tomatoes, croutons, Parmesan cheese, avocado slices, and flaked salmon.

In a small bowl, whisk together Greek yogurt, lemon juice, olive oil, salt, and pepper to create the dressing.

Before serving, gently toss the salad with the dressing after pouring it over it

Prep Time: 25 minutes

These heart-healthy salads are not only delicious but also provide a variety of nutrients to support your overall well-being. Enjoy experimenting with these recipes and adapting them to your taste preferences.

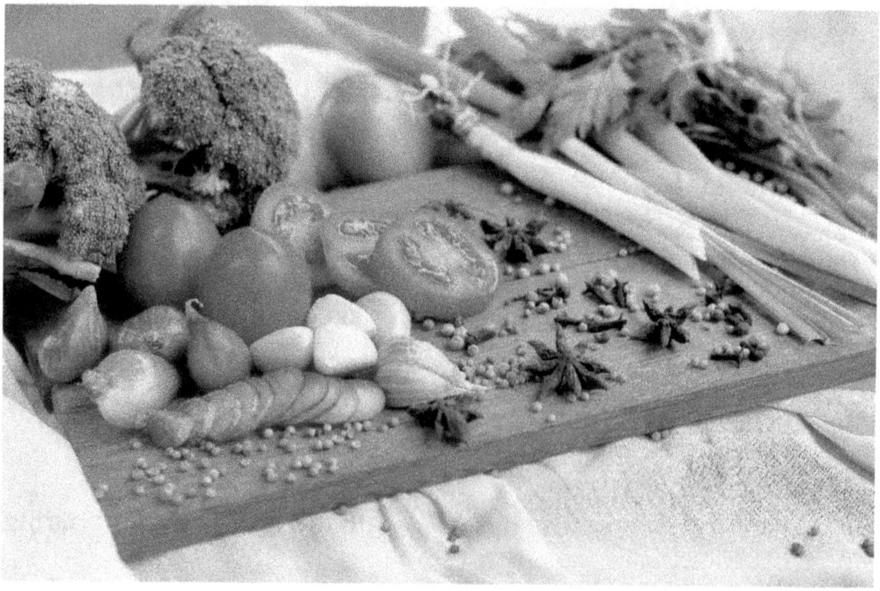

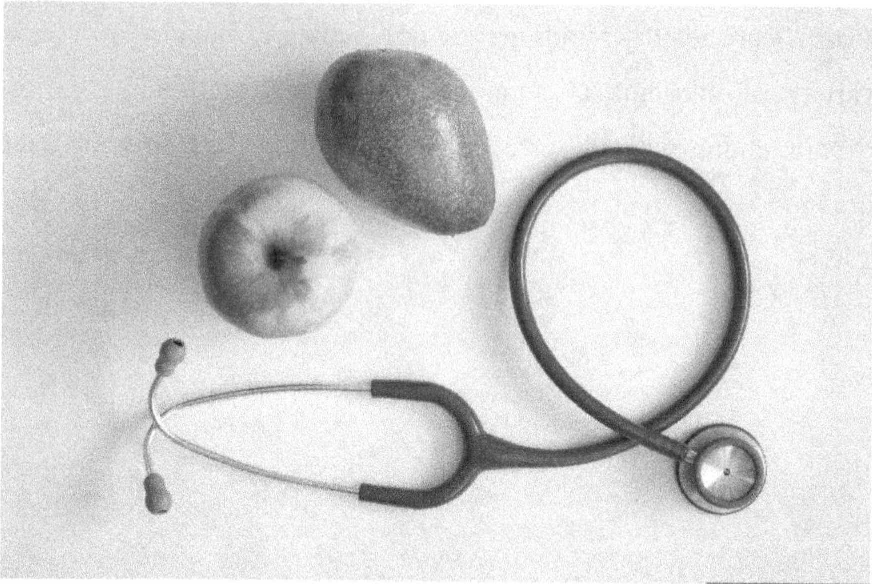

CHAPTER 4

Vegetable recipes

1. Grilled Veggie Skewers

Introduction:

Grilled Veggie Skewers are a delicious and heart-healthy way to enjoy a variety of colorful vegetables. Packed with antioxidants and fiber, this dish is a perfect addition to your heart-conscious diet.

Ingredients:

Bell peppers (red, yellow, green)

Cherry tomatoes

Zucchini

Red onion

Mushrooms

Olive oil

Garlic powder

Black pepper

Wooden skewers

Instructions:

Soak wooden skewers in water.

Chop vegetables into bite-sized pieces.

Thread veggies onto skewers.

Brush with olive oil and sprinkle with garlic powder and black pepper.

Grill until veggies are tender.

Serve hot.

Prep Time: 20 minutes

2. Quinoa Stuffed Bell Peppers

Introduction:

Quinoa Stuffed Bell Peppers are a nutrient-packed, heart-healthy delight. Quinoa provides protein, while bell peppers offer a rich source of vitamins. This colorful dish is both delicious and good for your heart.

Ingredients:

Bell peppers

Quinoa

Black beans

Corn

Tomatoes

Onion

Garlic

Cumin

Paprika

Low-sodium vegetable broth

Instructions:

Cook quinoa in vegetable broth.

Sauté onion and garlic, add tomatoes, black beans, corn, and spices.

Mix quinoa with the vegetable mixture.

Cut bell peppers in half, remove seeds.

Stuff peppers with quinoa mixture.

Bake until peppers are tender.

Prep Time: 40 minutes

3. Roasted Garlic Broccoli

Introduction:

Roasted Garlic Broccoli is a simple yet flavorful side dish. Broccoli is high in fiber and antioxidants, and roasting with garlic adds heart-healthy benefits. An easy and delicious side dish for any meal.

Ingredients:

Broccoli florets

Olive oil

Garlic cloves (minced)

Lemon juice

Salt and pepper

Instructions:

Toss broccoli with olive oil, minced garlic, and lemon juice.

Sprinkle with salt and pepper and spread out onto a baking sheet

Roast until broccoli is tender and edges are crispy.

Serve hot.

Prep Time: 25 minutes

4. Spinach and Chickpea Salad

Introduction:

This Spinach and Chickpea Salad is a power-packed meal. Spinach provides iron, while chickpeas offer protein and fiber. Combined with a light vinaigrette, it's a heart-healthy choice.

Ingredients:

Fresh spinach

Chickpeas (canned, drained)

Cherry tomatoes

Cucumber

Red onion

Feta cheese

Olive oil

Balsamic vinegar

Dijon mustard

Honey

Salt and pepper

Instructions:

Mix spinach, chickpeas, tomatoes, cucumber, red onion, and feta in a bowl.

In a separate bowl, whisk olive oil, balsamic vinegar, Dijon mustard, honey, salt, and pepper.

Drizzle the vinaigrette over the salad.

Toss gently and serve.

Prep Time: 15 minutes

5. Sweet Potato and Kale Hash

Introduction:

Sweet Potato and Kale Hash is a nutrient-dense breakfast option. Sweet potatoes are rich in vitamins, and kale adds an extra dose of antioxidants. This hearty dish will kickstart your day on a heart-healthy note.

Ingredients:

Sweet potatoes

Kale

Red onion

Garlic

Olive oil

Paprika

Cayenne pepper

Eggs (optional)

Instructions:

Dice sweet potatoes and sauté with olive oil, red onion, and garlic until tender.

Add chopped kale, paprika, and cayenne pepper.

Cook until kale is wilted.

Optionally, top with fried or poached eggs.

Prep Time: 30 minutes

6. Mediterranean Chickpea Salad

Introduction:

Mediterranean Chickpea Salad is a refreshing and heart-healthy dish. Chickpeas provide plant-based protein, and the colorful veggies add vitamins and minerals. The olive oil-based dressing is rich in healthy fats.

Ingredients:

Chickpeas (canned, drained)

Cucumber

Cherry tomatoes

Red bell pepper

Red onion

Kalamata olives

Feta cheese

Olive oil

Red wine vinegar

Dried oregano

Salt and pepper

Instructions:

Combine chickpeas, cucumber, tomatoes, bell pepper, red onion, olives, and feta in a bowl.

In a separate bowl, whisk olive oil, red wine vinegar, oregano, salt, and pepper.

Drizzle the salad with the dressing and carefully toss.

Serve chilled.

Prep Time: 20 minutes

7. Baked Eggplant Parmesan

Introduction:

Baked Eggplant Parmesan is a heart-healthy twist on a classic. Eggplant slices replace traditional fried cutlets, reducing saturated fat. This dish is a satisfying and flavorful option for a wholesome meal.

Ingredients:

Eggplant

Whole wheat breadcrumbs

Parmesan cheese

Mozzarella cheese

Marinara sauce (low sodium)

Egg whites

Fresh basil

Olive oil spray

Instructions:

Preheat oven and slice eggplant.

Dip eggplant slices in egg whites, coat with breadcrumbs.

Bake until golden.

Layer eggplant with marinara, mozzarella, and Parmesan.

Repeat layers and bake until cheese is melted and bubbly.

Garnish with fresh basil.

Prep Time: 45 minutes

8. Cauliflower Rice Stir-Fry

Introduction:

Cauliflower Rice Stir-Fry is a low-carb, heart-healthy alternative to traditional fried rice. Packed with colorful veggies and lean protein, this dish is both nutritious and delicious.

Ingredients:

Cauliflower (riced)

Mixed vegetables (bell peppers, carrots, peas)

Shrimp or tofu

Soy sauce (low sodium)

Sesame oil

Garlic

Ginger

Green onions

Eggs (optional)

Instructions:

Stir-fry shrimp or tofu until cooked.

Add garlic, ginger, and vegetables.

Push veggies to the side, scramble eggs if using.

Mix in cauliflower rice, soy sauce, and sesame oil.

Cook until heated through.

Garnish with green onions.

Prep Time: 30 minutes

9. Butternut Squash Soup

Introduction:

Butternut Squash Soup is a velvety, heart-healthy soup rich in vitamins and antioxidants. The natural sweetness of butternut squash combined with savory spices makes this a comforting and nutritious meal.

Ingredients:

Butternut squash

Onion

Carrots

Garlic

Vegetable broth (low sodium)

Coconut milk (light)

Ground nutmeg

Ground cinnamon

Salt and pepper

Instructions:

Peel and dice butternut squash, onions, and carrots.

Sauté onions and garlic until softened.

Add butternut squash, carrots, vegetable broth, and spices.

Simmer until vegetables are tender.

Blend the soup until smooth.

Stir in coconut milk.

Season with salt and pepper.

Reheat if necessary before serving.

Prep Time: 45 minutes

10. Zucchini Noodles with Pesto

Introduction:

Zucchini Noodles with Pesto is a low-carb alternative to pasta, offering a heart-healthy, flavorful option. Packed with fresh vegetables and a homemade pesto sauce, it's a light yet satisfying dish.

Ingredients:

Zucchini

Cherry tomatoes

Pesto sauce (fresh basil, pine nuts, garlic, Parmesan, olive oil)

Lemon zest

Salt and pepper

Instructions:

Spiralize zucchini into noodles.

Sauté zucchini noodles until just tender.

Toss with halved cherry tomatoes.

In a food processor, blend basil, pine nuts, garlic, Parmesan, and olive oil for pesto.

Mix pesto with zucchini noodles.

Zest the lemon and season with salt and pepper.

Serve immediately.

Prep Time: 25 minutes

These heart-healthy vegetable recipes are not only good for your cardiovascular health but also delicious and satisfying. You are welcome to alter them to suit your dietary requirements and tastes. Enjoy a variety of colorful, nutrient-packed meals to support your heart and overall well-being.

CHAPTER 5

Sauce and Stew Recipes

1. Classic Tomato Basil Marinara Sauce

Introduction: This heart-healthy tomato basil marinara sauce is a staple in Italian cuisine. Packed with antioxidants and low in saturated fats, it's a delicious and nutritious option for various dishes.

Ingredients:

2 tbsp olive oil

1 onion, finely chopped

3 garlic cloves, minced

28 oz crushed tomatoes

1 tsp dried oregano

1 tsp dried basil

Salt and pepper to taste

Instructions:

Heat olive oil in a saucepan, sauté onions until translucent.

Add garlic and cook for 1 minute.

Add the smashed tomatoes, salt, pepper, oregano, and basil

Simmer for 20-30 minutes, stirring occasionally.

Prep Time: 10 minutes

Heart-Health Benefits: Rich in lycopene and low in saturated fats.

2. Mediterranean Chickpea Stew

Introduction: This Mediterranean chickpea stew is a hearty, plant-based option loaded with fiber and heart-healthy ingredients.

Ingredients:

2 tbsp olive oil

1 onion, diced

3 carrots, sliced

2 zucchinis, diced

1 can chickpeas, drained

1 can diced tomatoes

3 cups vegetable broth

1 tsp cumin

1 tsp paprika

Salt and pepper to taste

Instructions:

Heat olive oil, sauté onions, carrots, and zucchinis.

Add chickpeas, diced tomatoes, vegetable broth, cumin, paprika, salt, and pepper.

Simmer for 25-30 minutes.

Prep Time: 15 minutes

Heart-Health Benefits: High fiber content and low in saturated fats.

3. Ginger-Turmeric Carrot Soup

Introduction: This ginger-turmeric carrot soup is not only comforting but also boasts anti-inflammatory properties, making it an excellent choice for heart health.

Ingredients:

2 tbsp olive oil

1 onion, chopped

1 lb carrots, peeled and sliced

1 tbsp fresh ginger, grated

1 tsp ground turmeric

4 cups vegetable broth

Salt and pepper to taste

Instructions:

Sauté onions in olive oil until soft, add carrots, ginger, and turmeric.

Pour in vegetable broth, bring to a boil, then simmer for 20 minutes.

Blend until smooth, season with salt and pepper.

Prep Time: 20 minutes

Heart-Health Benefits: Anti-inflammatory properties and low in saturated fats.

4. Spinach and White Bean Stew

Introduction: Packed with leafy greens and protein-rich white beans, this stew is a nutrient-dense option for a heart-healthy meal.

Ingredients:

2 tbsp olive oil

3 cloves garlic, minced

1 onion, diced

1 can white beans, drained

4 cups vegetable broth

6 cups fresh spinach

1 tsp dried thyme

Salt and pepper to taste

Instructions:

Add the onions and garlic to olive oil and sauté until aromatic

Add white beans, vegetable broth, spinach, thyme, salt, and pepper.

Simmer for 15-20 minutes.

Prep Time: 15 minutes

Heart-Health Benefits: High in fiber and low in saturated fats.

5. Lentil and Vegetable Curry

Introduction: This lentil and vegetable curry is a flavorful, plant-based option rich in fiber and heart-healthy nutrients.

Ingredients:

2 tbsp coconut oil

1 onion, chopped

2 carrots, sliced

1 cup dry lentils, rinsed

1 can coconut milk

2 tbsp curry powder

1 tsp turmeric

Salt and pepper to taste

Instructions:

Sauté onions and carrots in coconut oil until softened.

Add lentils, coconut milk, curry powder, turmeric, salt, and pepper.

Simmer for 25-30 minutes.

Prep Time: 20 minutes

Heart-Health Benefits: High fiber content and rich in plant-based proteins.

6. Roasted Red Pepper and Quinoa Soup

Introduction: Packed with the goodness of quinoa and roasted red peppers, this soup is a nutritious and heart-healthy option.

Ingredients:

2 tbsp olive oil

2 onions, diced

2 red bell peppers, roasted and chopped

1 cup quinoa, rinsed

6 cups vegetable broth

1 tsp smoked paprika

Salt and pepper to taste

Instructions:

Sauté onions in olive oil until translucent.

Add roasted red peppers, quinoa, vegetable broth, smoked paprika, salt, and pepper.

Simmer for 20-25 minutes.

Prep Time: 15 minutes

Heart-Health Benefits: Rich in quinoa, low in saturated fats.

7. Salmon and Vegetable Stew

Introduction: This hearty stew combines omega-3-rich salmon with a variety of vegetables for a heart-healthy and delicious meal.

Ingredients:

2 tbsp olive oil

4 salmon fillets

1 onion, diced

2 carrots, sliced

2 celery stalks, chopped

4 cups vegetable broth

1 tsp dill

Salt and pepper to taste

Instructions:

Sear salmon fillets in olive oil until golden, set aside.

Sauté onions, carrots, and celery until softened.

Add vegetable broth, dill, salt, and pepper. Simmer for 15-20 minutes.

Flake salmon into the stew before serving.

Prep Time: 25 minutes

Heart-Health Benefits: Omega-3 fatty acids from salmon.

8. Quinoa and Black Bean Chili

Introduction: This quinoa and black bean chili is a protein-packed, heart-healthy alternative to traditional meat-based chili.

Ingredients:

2 tbsp olive oil

1 onion, diced

2 bell peppers, diced

1 cup quinoa, rinsed

2 cans black beans, drained

1 can diced tomatoes

4 cups vegetable broth

2 tbsp chili powder

Salt and pepper to taste

Instructions:

Sauté onions and bell peppers in olive oil until tender.

Add quinoa, black beans, diced tomatoes, vegetable broth, chili powder, salt, and pepper.

Simmer for 20-25 minutes.

Prep Time: 20 minutes

Heart-Health Benefits: High fiber content and low in saturated fats.

9. Sweet Potato and Kale Stew

Introduction: Loaded with antioxidants from sweet potatoes and kale, this stew is a nutrient-dense and heart-healthy option.

Ingredients:

2 tbsp olive oil

1 onion, diced

3 sweet potatoes, peeled and cubed

4 cups vegetable broth

One bundle of chopped kale greens with the stems removed

1 tsp smoked paprika

Salt and pepper to taste

Instructions:

Sauté onions in olive oil until translucent.

Add sweet potatoes, vegetable broth, kale, smoked paprika, salt, and pepper.

Simmer for 25-30 minutes until sweet potatoes are tender.

Prep Time: 20 minutes

Heart-Health Benefits: Rich in vitamins, antioxidants, and low in saturated fats.

10. Turkey and Vegetable Stir-Fry

Introduction: A heart-healthy twist on a classic stir-fry, this recipe features lean turkey and a colorful array of vegetables.

Ingredients:

2 tbsp canola oil

1 lb lean ground turkey

1 broccoli head, florets separated

1 bell pepper, thinly sliced

1 zucchini, sliced

2 carrots, julienned

3 tbsp low-sodium soy sauce

1 tbsp honey

1 tsp ginger, grated

2 cloves garlic, minced

Instructions:

In a big skillet or wok, heat canola oil.

Brown ground turkey until fully cooked.

Add broccoli, bell pepper, zucchini, and carrots. Stir-fry until vegetables are tender-crisp.

Combine the soy sauce, honey, garlic, and ginger in a small bowl. Pour over the turkey and vegetables, toss to coat.

Cook for an additional 2-3 minutes.

Prep Time: 25 minutes

Heart-Health Benefits: Lean protein from turkey, low in saturated fats.

These recipes provide a variety of delicious options for heart-healthy sauces and stews. Remember to consult with a healthcare professional or a nutritionist for personalized dietary advice.

CHAPTER 6

Vegetarian Recipes

1. Quinoa-Stuffed Bell Peppers

Introduction:

These Quinoa-Stuffed Bell Peppers are a delightful combination of protein-packed quinoa, colorful vegetables, and heart-healthy spices. Packed with nutrients and flavor, they make for a satisfying and nutritious meal.

Ingredients:

4 large bell peppers (any color)

1 cup quinoa, cooked

One can (15 oz) of rinsed and drained black beans

1 cup corn kernels (fresh or frozen)

1 cup diced tomatoes

1 cup diced red onion

1 teaspoon cumin

1 teaspoon chili powder

Salt and pepper to taste

1 cup shredded low-fat cheese (optional)

Instructions:

Preheat the oven to 375°F (190°C).

Slice off the bell peppers' tops, then take out the seeds and membranes

In a large bowl, combine cooked quinoa, black beans, corn, tomatoes, red onion, cumin, chili powder, salt, and pepper.

Stuff the quinoa mixture inside each bell pepper.

Place the stuffed peppers in a baking dish, and optionally, sprinkle shredded cheese on top.

Bake the peppers for 25 to 30 minutes, or until they are soft

Serve warm and enjoy!

Prep Time: 15 minutes | **Cook Time:** 30 minutes

2. Mushroom and Spinach Lentil Loaf

Introduction:

This Mushroom and Spinach Lentil Loaf is a hearty and heart-healthy alternative to traditional meatloaf. Packed with fiber and nutrients, it's a flavorful dish that's perfect for a wholesome dinner.

Ingredients:

2 cups cooked green lentils

1 cup finely chopped mushrooms

1 cup chopped spinach

1/2 cup oats

1/2 cup breadcrumbs

1 onion, finely chopped

2 cloves garlic, minced

2 tablespoons tomato paste

1 teaspoon dried thyme

1 teaspoon smoked paprika

Salt and pepper to taste

Instructions:

Preheat the oven to 375°F (190°C).

In a pan, sauté mushrooms, spinach, onion, and garlic until softened.

In a large bowl, combine lentils, sautéed vegetables, oats, breadcrumbs, tomato paste, thyme, smoked paprika, salt, and pepper.

Transfer the mixture to a loaf pan, pressing it down evenly.

Bake for 45 to 60 minutes, or until golden brown on top.

Allow it to cool slightly before slicing.

Prep Time: 20 minutes | Cook Time: 45 minutes

3. Chickpea and Vegetable Stir-Fry

Introduction:

This Chickpea and Vegetable Stir-Fry is a quick and easy recipe that's rich in plant-based protein and heart-healthy ingredients. Bursting with vibrant colors and flavors, it's a nutritious option for a speedy weeknight dinner.

Ingredients:

2 cans (15 oz each) chickpeas, drained and rinsed

3 cups of mixed veggies, including snap peas, bell peppers, and broccoli

1 cup sliced carrots

1/4 cup low-sodium soy sauce

2 tablespoons sesame oil

1 tablespoon ginger, minced

2 cloves garlic, minced

1 tablespoon maple syrup

1 tablespoon cornstarch

Sesame seeds for garnish (optional)

Instructions:

Sesame oil should be heated over medium-high heat in a wok or big skillet

Add ginger and garlic, stir-fry for 1 minute.

Add mixed vegetables and carrots, stir-fry until crisp-tender.

In a small bowl, whisk together soy sauce, maple syrup, and cornstarch.

Pour the sauce over the vegetables and add chickpeas, stirring until well-coated and heated through.

Garnish with sesame seeds if desired.

Serve over brown rice or quinoa.

Prep Time: 15 minutes | Cook Time: 15 minutes

4. Sweet Potato and Black Bean Chili

Introduction:

This Sweet Potato and Black Bean Chili is a satisfying and nutritious option for chilly days. Packed with fiber, vitamins, and minerals, it's a flavorful bowl of goodness that's gentle on the heart.

Ingredients:

2 medium sweet potatoes, peeled and diced

One can (15 oz) of rinsed and drained black beans

1 can (14 oz) diced tomatoes

1 onion, chopped

2 cloves garlic, minced

1 bell pepper, diced

2 teaspoons chili powder

1 teaspoon cumin

1/2 teaspoon smoked paprika

Salt and pepper to taste

4 cups vegetable broth

1 tablespoon olive oil

Instructions:

Warm up the olive oil in a big pot over medium heat. Add onion, garlic, and bell pepper, sauté until softened.

Add sweet potatoes, black beans, diced tomatoes, chili powder, cumin, smoked paprika, salt, and pepper.

After adding the vegetable broth, boil the mixture.

Cover and cook for 20-25 minutes or until sweet potatoes are tender.

Adjust seasoning if needed and serve hot.

Prep Time: 15 minutes | Cook Time: 25 minutes

5. Mediterranean Chickpea Salad

Introduction:

This Mediterranean Chickpea Salad is a refreshing and heart-healthy dish featuring the vibrant flavors of the Mediterranean. Packed with fiber, antioxidants, and good fats, it's perfect as a light lunch or a side dish.

Ingredients:

2 cans (15 oz each) chickpeas, drained and rinsed

1 cucumber, diced

1 cup cherry tomatoes, halved

1/2 cup Kalamata olives, sliced

1/2 cup red onion, finely chopped

1/2 cup feta cheese, crumbled

1/4 cup extra-virgin olive oil

2 tablespoons red wine vinegar

1 teaspoon dried oregano

Salt and pepper to taste

Fresh parsley for garnish

Instructions:

In a large bowl, combine chickpeas, cucumber, cherry tomatoes, olives, red onion, and feta cheese.

In a small bowl, whisk together olive oil, red wine vinegar, dried oregano, salt, and pepper.

After adding the dressing to the salad, stir to fully incorporate

Garnish with fresh parsley.

Let it cool for a minimum of half an hour before serving.

Prep Time: 15 minutes | Chill Time: 30 minutes

6. Lentil and Vegetable Curry

Introduction:

This Lentil and Vegetable Curry is a fragrant and heart-healthy dish that's rich in plant-based proteins. Bursting with aromatic spices and colorful vegetables, it's a comforting option for a wholesome dinner.

Ingredients:

1 cup dry brown lentils, rinsed

1 can (14 oz) coconut milk

1 onion, finely chopped

2 cloves garlic, minced

1 bell pepper, diced

1 zucchini, diced

1 carrot, sliced

2 tablespoons curry powder

1 teaspoon turmeric

1 teaspoon cumin

1/2 teaspoon coriander

Salt and pepper to taste

2 tablespoons olive oil

Fresh cilantro for garnish

Instructions:

Warm up the olive oil in a big pot over medium heat. Add onion and garlic, sauté until softened.

Add curry powder, turmeric, cumin, and coriander. Stir to coat the onions and garlic in the spices.

Add lentils, coconut milk, bell pepper, zucchini, and carrot. Season with salt and pepper.

Once the lentils are tender, simmer for 25 to 30 minutes on low heat after bringing to a boil

Adjust seasoning if needed.

Serve over brown rice or quinoa and garnish with fresh cilantro.

Prep Time: 15 minutes | Cook Time: 30 minutes

7. Spinach and Feta Stuffed Portobello Mushrooms

Introduction:

These Spinach and Feta Stuffed Portobello Mushrooms are a savory delight, combining the earthy flavors of mushrooms with the richness of spinach and feta. A delicious and heart-healthy option for a light dinner or appetizer.

Ingredients:

4 large Portobello mushrooms, stems removed

2 cups fresh spinach, chopped

1 cup crumbled feta cheese

1/4 cup grated Parmesan cheese

2 cloves garlic, minced

2 tablespoons olive oil

Salt and pepper to taste

Fresh parsley for garnish

Instructions:

Preheat the oven to 375°F (190°C).

Heat the olive oil in a pan over medium heat. Add garlic and sauté until fragrant.

Add chopped spinach and cook until wilted.

In a bowl, combine spinach, feta, Parmesan, salt, and pepper.

Place Portobello mushrooms on a baking sheet and fill each with the spinach and feta mixture.

Bake for 20-25 minutes or until mushrooms are tender.

Garnish with fresh parsley before serving.

Prep Time: 15 minutes | Cook Time: 25 minutes

8. Broccoli and Chickpea Quinoa Bowl

Introduction:

This Broccoli and Chickpea Quinoa Bowl is a nutrient-packed powerhouse, combining the goodness of quinoa, chickpeas, and vibrant broccoli. It's a quick and easy recipe that's perfect for a satisfying lunch or dinner.

Ingredients:

1 cup quinoa, cooked

One can (15 oz) of rinsed and drained chickpeas

2 cups broccoli florets

1 bell pepper, thinly sliced

2 tablespoons olive oil

1 teaspoon garlic powder

1 teaspoon smoked paprika

Salt and pepper to taste

Juice of 1 lemon

1/4 cup chopped almonds (optional)

Instructions:

Heat the olive oil in a big skillet over medium heat

Add chickpeas, broccoli, and bell pepper to the skillet. Sprinkle with garlic powder, smoked paprika, salt, and pepper.

Sauté until the vegetables are tender and chickpeas are golden brown.

In a bowl, combine cooked quinoa and the sautéed mixture.

Squeeze lemon juice over the bowl and toss to combine.

Garnish with chopped almonds if desired.

Prep Time: 15 minutes | Cook Time: 15 minutes

9. Cauliflower and Chickpea Coconut Curry

Introduction:

This Cauliflower and Chickpea Coconut Curry is a creamy and flavorful dish that's both comforting and heart-healthy. Packed with vegetables and spices, it's a satisfying option for a wholesome dinner.

Ingredients:

1 small head cauliflower, cut into florets

One can (15 oz) of rinsed and drained chickpeas

1 can (14 oz) coconut milk

1 onion, finely chopped

2 cloves garlic, minced

1 tablespoon curry powder

1 teaspoon turmeric

1 teaspoon cumin

1/2 teaspoon coriander

Salt and pepper to taste

2 tablespoons olive oil

Fresh cilantro for garnish

Instructions:

Warm up the olive oil in a big pot over medium heat. Add onion and garlic, sauté until softened.

Add curry powder, turmeric, cumin, and coriander. Stir to coat the onions and garlic in the spices.

Add cauliflower, chickpeas, and coconut milk. Season with salt and pepper.

Bring to a boil, then reduce heat and simmer for 20-25 minutes or until cauliflower is tender.

Adjust seasoning if needed.

Add fresh cilantro as a garnish and serve over brown rice.

Prep Time: 15 minutes | Cook Time: 25 minutes

10. **Avocado and Black Bean Quinoa Salad**

Introduction:

This Avocado and Black Bean Quinoa Salad is a refreshing and heart-healthy option for a light lunch or side dish. Packed with protein, fiber, and healthy fats, it's a delicious way to nourish your body.

Ingredients:

1 cup quinoa, cooked

One can (15 oz) of rinsed and drained black beans

1 avocado, diced

1 cup cherry tomatoes, halved

1/4 cup red onion, finely chopped

1/4 cup fresh cilantro, chopped

Juice of 2 limes

2 tablespoons olive oil

Salt and pepper to taste

Instructions:

In a large bowl, combine cooked quinoa, black beans, avocado, cherry tomatoes, red onion, and cilantro.

Mix the lime juice, olive oil, salt, and pepper in a small bowl.

After adding the dressing to the salad, stir to fully incorporate.

Let it cool for a minimum of half an hour before serving

Prep Time: 15 minutes | Chill Time: 30 minutes

These heart-healthy vegetarian recipes are not only nutritious but also delicious, providing a variety of flavors and textures to keep your meals exciting and satisfying.

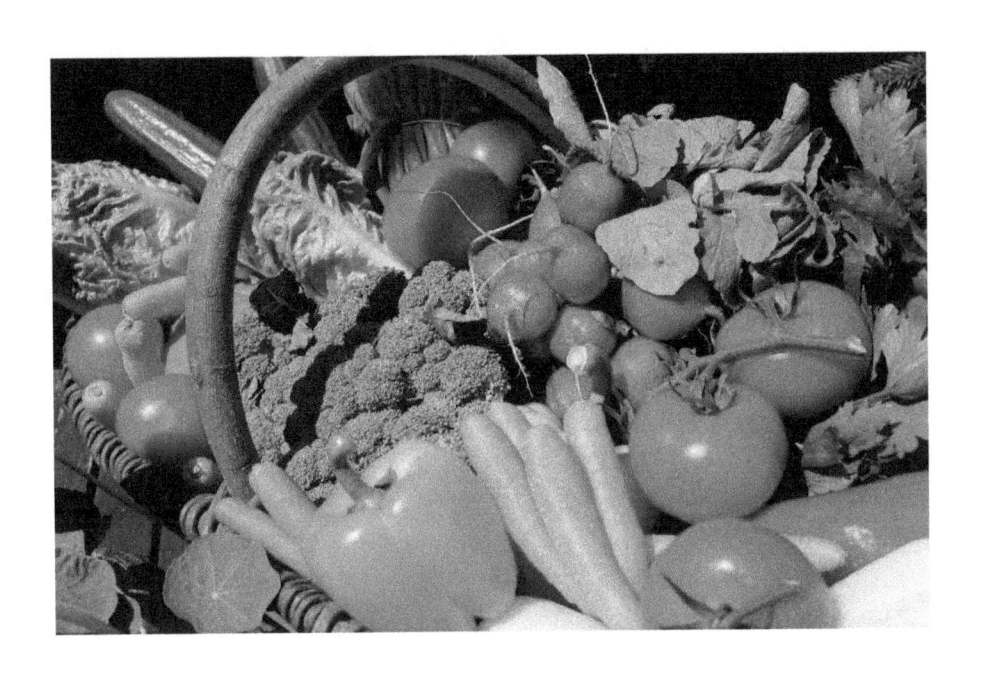

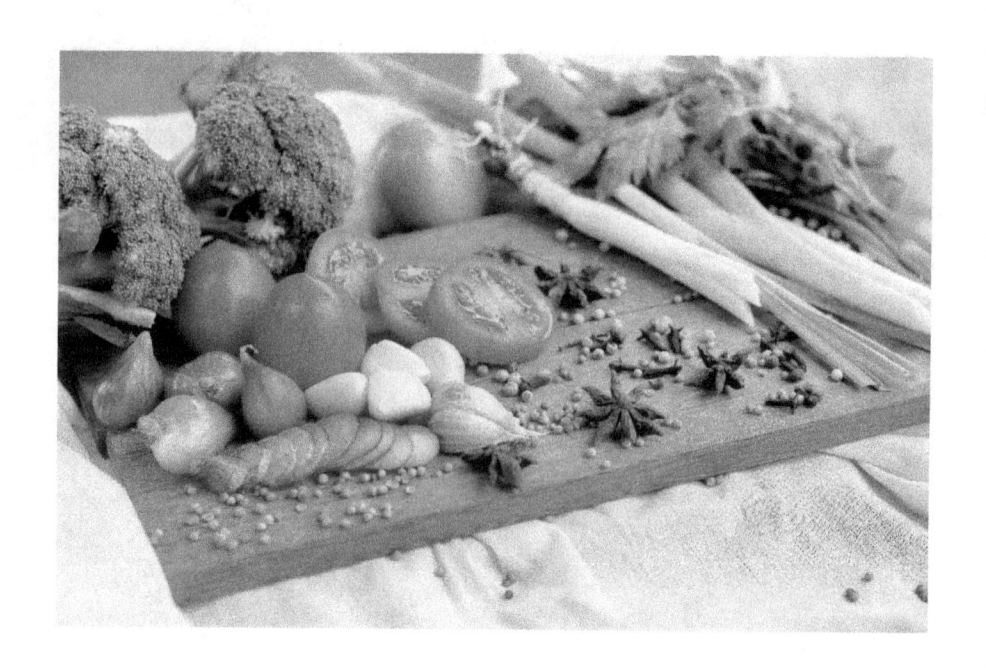

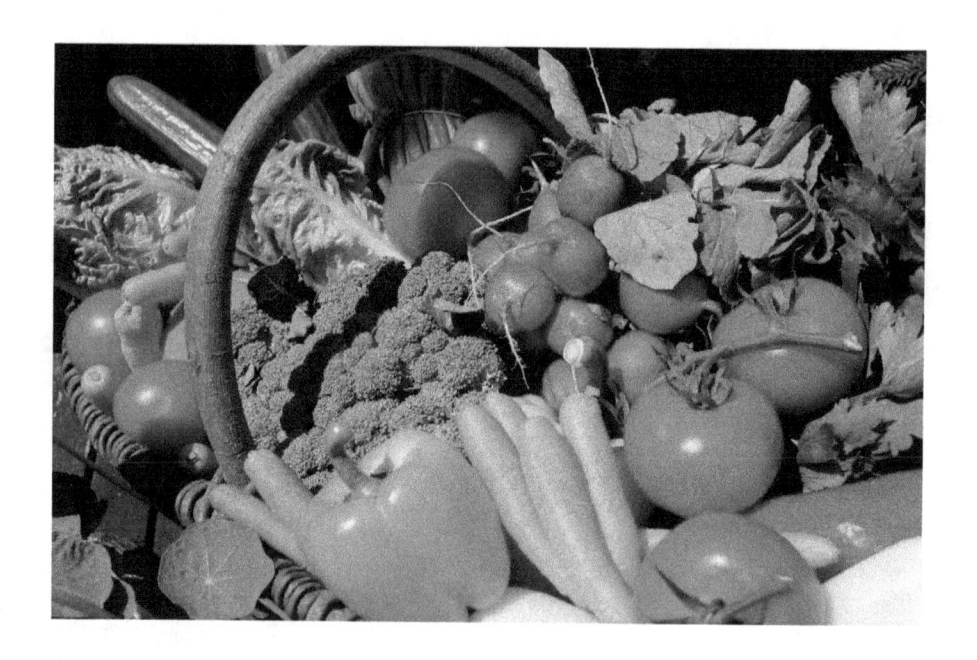

CHAPTER 7

Snacks and Desserts Recipes

Snacks:

1. Roasted Chickpeas:

Ingredients:

One can (15 oz) of rinsed and drained chickpeas

1 tablespoon olive oil

1 teaspoon smoked paprika

1/2 teaspoon cumin

1/2 teaspoon garlic powder

Salt to taste

Instructions:

Preheat oven to 400°F (200°C).

Pat chickpeas dry and toss with olive oil and spices.

Place on a baking sheet, then bake until crispy, 20 to 25 minutes.

2. Greek Yogurt Parfait:

Ingredients:

1 cup low-fat Greek yogurt

1/2 cup mixed berries

2 tablespoons chopped nuts (almonds or walnuts)

1 tablespoon honey

Instructions:

In a glass, layer Greek yogurt, berries, and nuts.

Drizzle honey on top. Repeat layers.

3. Veggie Sticks with Hummus:

Ingredients:

Carrot, cucumber, and bell pepper sticks

Hummus (store-bought or homemade)

Instructions:

Cut vegetables into sticks.

Serve with a side of hummus for a crunchy, satisfying snack.

4. Baked Sweet Potato Chips:

Ingredients:

2 sweet potatoes, thinly sliced

1 tablespoon olive oil

1/2 teaspoon sea salt

Instructions:

Preheat oven to 375°F (190°C).

Toss sweet potato slices with olive oil and salt.

Bake for 15-20 minutes until crisp.

5. Edamame with Sea Salt:

Ingredients:

2 cups edamame (fresh or frozen)

Sea salt to taste

Instructions:

Boil or steam edamame until tender.

Sprinkle with sea salt and enjoy!

Desserts:

6. Berry Chia Seed Pudding:

Ingredients:

1/4 cup chia seeds

1 cup almond milk

1/2 teaspoon vanilla extract

Mixed berries for topping

Instructions:

Mix chia seeds, almond milk, and vanilla. Refrigerate overnight.

Top with fresh berries before serving.

7. Dark Chocolate-Dipped Strawberries:

Ingredients:

1 cup dark chocolate chips

1 pint strawberries, washed and dried

Instructions:

Melt chocolate in a microwave-safe bowl.

Dip each strawberry into melted chocolate. Allow to cool.

8. Baked Apples with Cinnamon:

Ingredients:

4 apples, cored and halved

1 teaspoon cinnamon

1 tablespoon honey

Instructions:

Preheat oven to 375°F (190°C).

Sprinkle apples with cinnamon and drizzle with honey. Bake until tender.

9. Frozen Banana Bites:

Ingredients:

Bananas, sliced

Greek yogurt

Nuts or seeds for coating

Instructions:

Dip banana slices in yogurt, coat with nuts or seeds.

Freeze until firm.

10. Oatmeal Raisin Energy Bites:

Ingredients:

1 cup rolled oats

1/2 cup almond butter

1/4 cup honey

1/2 cup raisins

Instructions:

Mix all ingredients, roll into bite-sized balls.

Let it cool for a minimum of half an hour before serving.

These snacks and desserts are not only delicious but also rich in nutrients that support heart health. To fit your dietary requirements, adjust the portion quantities.

CHAPTER 8

Smoothies Recipes

1. Berry Blast Smoothie:

Ingredients:

1 cup mixed berries (strawberries, blueberries, raspberries)

1/2 banana

1/2 cup Greek yogurt (low-fat)

1 tablespoon chia seeds

1 cup spinach

1 cup almond milk

Instructions:

Blend all ingredients until smooth.

Add ice if desired.

2. Green Power Smoothie:

Ingredients:

1 cup kale (stems removed)

1/2 cucumber

1/2 avocado

1/2 lemon (juiced)

1 tablespoon flaxseeds

1 cup coconut water

Instructions:

Blend all ingredients until creamy.

Adjust consistency with more coconut water if needed.

3. **Heart-Healthy Citrus Smoothie:**

Ingredients:

1 orange (peeled)

1/2 cup pineapple chunks

1/2 cup mango chunks

1 tablespoon hemp seeds

1 cup Greek yogurt (low-fat)

Ice cubes

Instructions:

Blend all ingredients until smooth.

Serve over ice.

4. Antioxidant-Packed Smoothie:

Ingredients:

1 cup mixed berries (blueberries, raspberries, blackberries)

1/2 cup pomegranate seeds

1/2 banana

1 tablespoon walnuts

1 cup spinach

1 cup almond milk

Instructions:

Blend until well combined.

Garnish with extra berries and nuts.

5. Heart-Boosting Beet Smoothie:

Ingredients:

1 small cooked beet (peeled and cubed)

1/2 cup strawberries

1/2 cup raspberries

1/2 cup Greek yogurt (low-fat)

1 tablespoon chia seeds

1 cup coconut water

Instructions:

Blend until the mixture is smooth.

Adjust sweetness with honey if needed.

6. Almond Butter Banana Smoothie:

Ingredients:

1 banana

2 tablespoons almond butter

1/2 cup rolled oats

1/2 teaspoon cinnamon

1 cup almond milk

Ice cubes

Instructions:

Blend until creamy.

Top with a sprinkle of cinnamon.

7. Cherry Almond Delight:

Ingredients:

1 cup cherries (pitted)

1/2 cup plain Greek yogurt

1/4 cup almonds

1 tablespoon flaxseeds

1 cup almond milk

Instructions:

Blend until smooth.

Garnish with sliced almonds.

8. Mango Turmeric Smoothie:

Ingredients:

1 cup mango chunks

1/2 teaspoon turmeric

1/2 teaspoon ginger (freshly grated)

1 tablespoon chia seeds

1 cup coconut water

Instructions:

Blend until smooth.

Serve with a sprinkle of chia seeds on top.

9. **Cocoa Avocado Smoothie:**

Ingredients:

1/2 avocado

2 tablespoons cocoa powder (unsweetened)

1 tablespoon honey

1/2 teaspoon vanilla extract

1 cup almond milk

Instructions:

Blend until creamy.

Adjust sweetness as needed.

10. Peachy Keen Protein Smoothie:

Ingredients:

1 cup peaches (fresh or frozen)

1/2 cup cottage cheese

1/2 cup almond milk

1 tablespoon hemp seeds

1/2 teaspoon vanilla extract

Ice cubes

Instructions:

Blend until smooth and creamy.

Enjoy as a post-workout snack.

These heart-healthy smoothies are packed with nutrients and antioxidants to support cardiovascular health. Adjust ingredients to suit your taste preferences and dietary needs.

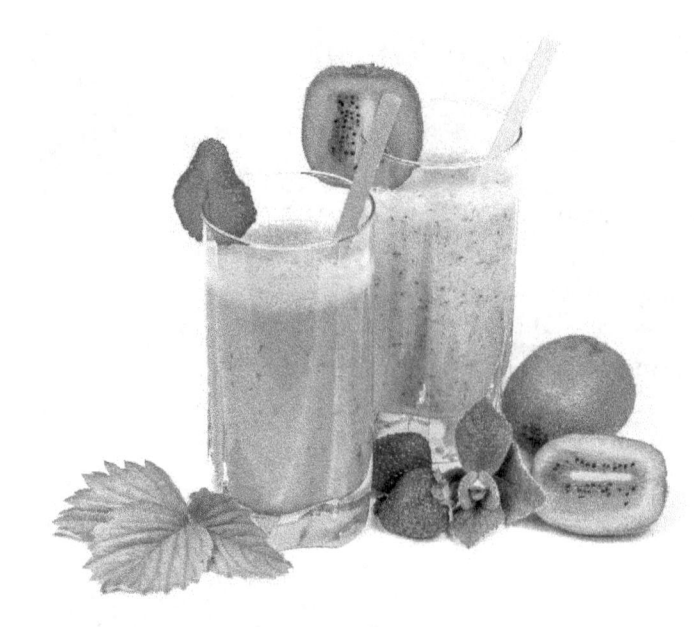

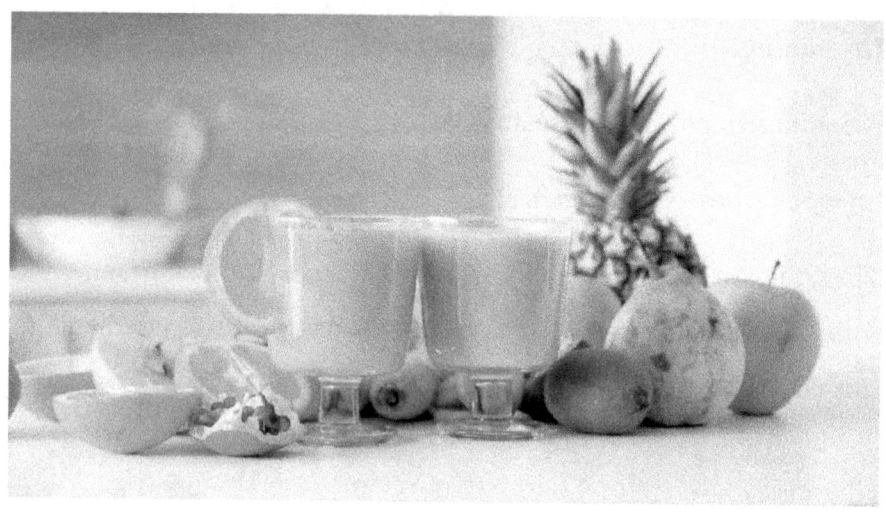

CHAPTER 9

30 Days Heart Healthy Meal Plan

Day 1:

Breakfast: Berries and chia seeds mixed into oatmeal

Lunch: Grilled chicken salad with mixed vegetables

Snack: Greek yogurt with sliced almonds

Dinner: Baked salmon with quinoa and steamed broccoli

Day 2:

Breakfast: Poached eggs and avocado on whole grain bread

Lunch would be healthy grain crackers on the side and lentil soup.

Snack: Fresh fruit (e.g., apple slices)

Dinner: Stir-fried tofu with brown rice and vegetables

Day 3:

Breakfast: Smoothie with spinach, banana, and berries

Lunch: Quinoa salad topped with cucumber, feta cheese, and chickpeas

Snack: Handful of nuts (e.g., walnuts or almonds)

Dinner: Grilled shrimp with sweet potato and asparagus

Day 4:

Breakfast: Greek yogurt parfait with granola and fresh fruit

Lunch: Turkey and vegetable whole grain wrap

Snack: Carrot and cucumber sticks with hummus

Dinner: Quinoa-topped baked chicken and roasted Brussels sprouts

Day 5:

Breakfast: Pancakes made with whole grains served with a side of mixed fruit

Lunch: Spinach and feta-stuffed chicken breast with quinoa

Snack: Cottage cheese with pineapple chunks

Dinner: Brown rice and green beans with baked fish

Day 6:

Breakfast: Slicing a banana and serving whole grain cereal with low-fat milk

Lunch: Vegetable and bean burrito bowl

Snack: Orange slices

Dinner: Stir-fried broccoli and tofu with brown rice

Day 7:

Breakfast: Spinach-filled scrambled eggs and wholegrain bread

Lunch: Chickpea and vegetable stir-fry

Snack: Handful of mixed berries

Dinner: Quinoa, grilled fish, and steamed asparagus

Day 8:

Breakfast: Overnight oats with almond butter and sliced strawberries

Lunch: Turkey and vegetable stir-fry with brown rice

Snack: Handful of cherry tomatoes

Dinner: Baked chicken breast with quinoa and roasted sweet potatoes

Day 9:

Breakfast: Whole grain bagel with smoked salmon and cream cheese

Lunch: Curry with lentils and veggies served over basmati rice

Snack: Apple slices with peanut butter

Dinner: Grilled shrimp skewers with quinoa and sautéed spinach

Day 10:

Breakfast: Avocado and tomato omelet with whole grain toast

Lunch: Black bean and quinoa salad dressed with a lime vinaigrette

Snack: Mixed nuts (e.g., almonds, pistachios)

Dinner: Baked cod with couscous and roasted zucchini

Day 11:

Breakfast: Whole grain waffles topped with a dollop of yogurt and fresh berries

Lunch is a Caesar salad made with grilled chicken and whole grain croutons.

Snack: Sliced cucumber with hummus

Dinner: Stir-fried tofu with brown rice and broccoli

Day 12:

Breakfast: Smoothie bowl with spinach, banana, and topped with granola

Lunch: Carrot sticks on the side and a sandwich with turkey and avocado

Snack: Cottage cheese with peach slices

Dinner: Salmon baked with sautéed kale and quinoa

Day 13:

Breakfast: Whole grain English muffin with scrambled eggs and tomato slices

Lunch: Chickpea and vegetable Buddha bowl

Snack: Orange slices with a handful of almonds

Dinner: Brussels sprouts with quinoa paired with grilled shrimp

Day 14:

Breakfast: Greek yogurt parfait topped with mixed berries, honey, and oats

Lunch: Spinach and feta-stuffed chicken breast with quinoa

Snack: Handful of walnuts and a small apple

Dinner: Baked cod with brown rice and steamed broccoli

Day 15:

Breakfast: Spinach-filled scrambled eggs and wholegrain bread

Lunch: Supper will be lentil soup and whole grain crackers.

Snack: Carrot and cucumber sticks with hummus

Dinner: Brussels sprouts and quinoa paired with grilled chicken

Day 16:

Breakfast: Overnight chia seed pudding with almond milk and sliced mango

Lunch: Turkey and vegetable stir-fry with brown rice

Snack: Orange slices with a handful of mixed nuts

Dinner: Baked salmon with sweet potato and asparagus

Day 17:

Breakfast: Whole grain bagel with smoked salmon, cream cheese, and tomato slices

Lunch: Black bean and quinoa salad dressed with a lime vinaigrette

Snack: Greek yogurt with sliced almonds and a drizzle of honey

Dinner: Grilled shrimp skewers with quinoa and sautéed spinach

Day 18:

Breakfast: Avocado and tomato omelet with whole grain toast

Lunch: Stir-fried vegetables and chickpeas over brown rice

Snack: Mixed berries with a small handful of pistachios

Dinner: Baked chicken breast with quinoa and roasted sweet potatoes

Day 19:

Breakfast: Smoothie bowl with spinach, banana, and topped with granola

Lunch: Carrot sticks on the side and a sandwich with turkey and avocado

Snack: Cottage cheese with peach slices

Dinner: Baked cod with couscous and roasted zucchini

Day 20:

Breakfast: Whole grain English muffin with scrambled eggs and tomato slices

Lunch: Caesar salad made with grilled chicken and whole grain croutons

Snack: Sliced cucumber with hummus

Dinner: Stir-fried tofu with brown rice and broccoli

Day 21:

Waffles made with whole grains, fresh berries, and a dollop of yogurt for breakfast.

Lunch consists of quinoa and grilled chicken and vegetable kebabs.

Snack: A spoonful of almond butter spread over some apple slices.

Dinner: Lentil and vegetable curry with brown rice

Day 22:

Breakfast: Greek yogurt smoothie with kale, banana, and berries

Lunch: Turkey and vegetable whole grain wrap

Snack: Handful of cherry tomatoes

Dinner: Grilled salmon with quinoa and sautéed kale

Day 23:

Breakfast: Overnight oats with almond butter and sliced strawberries

Lunch: Quinoa salad topped with cucumber, feta cheese, and chickpeas

Snack: Mixed nuts (e.g., walnuts, almonds)

Dinner: Quinoa-topped baked chicken and roasted Brussels sprouts

Day 24:

Breakfast: Poached eggs and avocado on whole grain bread

Lunch: Spinach and feta-stuffed chicken breast with quinoa

Snack: Carrot and celery sticks with hummus

Dinner: Baked cod with brown rice and steamed broccoli

Day 25:

Breakfast: Smoothie with spinach, banana, and berries

Lunch: Supper will be lentil soup and whole grain crackers.

Snack: Fresh fruit (e.g., apple slices)

Dinner: Stir-fried tofu with brown rice and vegetables

Day 26:

Breakfast: Greek yogurt parfait topped with mixed berries and granola

Lunch: Turkey and vegetable stir-fry with brown rice

Snack: Handful of nuts (e.g., walnuts or almonds)

Dinner: Grilled shrimp with quinoa and roasted sweet potatoes

Day 27:

Breakfast: Whole grain pancakes with a side of sliced peaches

Lunch: Chickpea and vegetable Buddha bowl

Snack: Cottage cheese with pineapple chunks

Dinner: Baked salmon with quinoa and asparagus

Day 28:

Breakfast consists of whole grain bread and scrambled eggs with spinach.

Lunch would be a lime vinaigrette black bean and quinoa salad

Snack: Handful of mixed berries

Dinner: Brown rice, roasted zucchini, and grilled shrimp

Day 29:

Breakfast: Whole grain bagel with smoked salmon and cream cheese

Lunch: Caesar salad made with grilled chicken and whole grain croutons

Snack: Sliced cucumber with hummus

Dinner: Stir-fried tofu with quinoa and sautéed spinach

Day 30:

Breakfast: Avocado and tomato omelet with whole grain toast

Lunch: Stir-fried vegetables and turkey over brown rice

Snack: Berries combined with a small amount of almonds

Dinner: Baked cod with couscous and roasted vegetables

CHAPTER 10

HEART HEALTHY FRUITS

Blueberries:

Introduction: Blueberries are vibrant, antioxidant-rich berries that come in various varieties, such as wild and cultivated.

Nutrients: Packed with anthocyanins, vitamin C, and fiber.

Heart Health Benefits: The antioxidants in blueberries have been linked to reduced blood pressure and improved cholesterol levels.

Avocado:

Introduction: Creamy and versatile, avocados are unique fruits known for their rich, monounsaturated fats.

Nutrients: High in healthy fats, potassium, and folate.

Heart Health Benefits: Avocados may help lower bad cholesterol (LDL) levels and support overall cardiovascular health.

Oranges:

Introduction: Oranges are juicy citrus fruits known for their refreshing taste and wide availability.

Nutrients: Rich in fiber, potassium, and vitamin C.

Heart Health Benefits: The potassium in oranges supports blood pressure regulation, while vitamin C acts as a powerful antioxidant.

Strawberries:

Introduction: Strawberries are sweet, red berries commonly enjoyed fresh or in various dishes.

Nutrients: Packed with antioxidants, manganese, and vitamin C.

Heart Health Benefits: Strawberries contribute to heart health by promoting healthy blood vessels and reducing inflammation.

Apples:

Introduction: Apples are crisp and sweet fruits that come in various varieties and colors.

Nutrients: High in fiber, vitamin C, and various antioxidants.

Heart Health Benefits: The soluble fiber in apples helps lower cholesterol levels and supports heart health.

Bananas:

Introduction: Bananas are convenient, potassium-rich fruits with a natural sweetness.

Nutrients: High in potassium, vitamin B6, and fiber.

Heart Health Benefits: Potassium in bananas helps regulate blood pressure and supports cardiovascular health.

Grapes:

Introduction: Grapes come in different colors and are often enjoyed fresh or as raisins.

Nutrients: Rich in antioxidants, including resveratrol, and vitamins like vitamin K and vitamin C.

Heart Health Benefits: Resveratrol in grapes is associated with improved heart health by promoting healthy blood vessels.

Pomegranates:

Introduction: Pomegranates are unique fruits filled with juicy, ruby-red seeds.

Nutrients: High in antioxidants, particularly punicalagins and anthocyanins.

Heart Health Benefits: Pomegranates may help lower blood pressure and reduce oxidative stress in the body.

Kiwi:

Introduction: Kiwi, with its fuzzy brown skin and vibrant green flesh, is a nutrient-dense fruit.

Nutrients: Rich in vitamin C, vitamin K, and dietary fiber.

Heart Health Benefits: Kiwi supports heart health by aiding in blood clotting and reducing blood pressure.

Cherries:

Introduction: Cherries, whether sweet or tart, are delicious fruits with a deep red hue.

Nutrients: Packed with antioxidants, including anthocyanins and quercetin.

Heart Health Benefits: Cherries may help reduce inflammation and lower risk factors for heart disease.

Incorporating a variety of these heart-healthy fruits into your diet can contribute to overall cardiovascular well-being. Remember to enjoy them as part of a balanced and varied diet alongside other heart-healthy foods.

CONCLUSION

The journey through the pages of this heart-healthy cookbook has been a flavorful exploration of not just delightful culinary creations, but also a commitment to nurturing a healthier heart and a vibrant life.

As we close the chapters of this culinary odyssey, it is evident that the power to safeguard our cardiovascular health lies not only in the hands of medical professionals but also in the choices we make daily in our kitchens.

Throughout these recipes, we've discovered the exquisite balance between taste and well-being. From vibrant salads bursting with antioxidants to hearty, wholesome grains and lean proteins, each dish has been crafted with the intention of promoting heart health without compromising on the joy of eating.

It is a testament to the idea that nourishing our bodies can be a celebration of both flavor and vitality.

The heart, a symbol of life and love, deserves our utmost care and attention. This cookbook stands as a culinary guide, offering a palette of ingredients and cooking techniques that not only satisfy our taste buds but also fortify our cardiovascular system.

By embracing the principles of mindful eating, portion control, and the incorporation of heart-friendly ingredients, we empower ourselves to make informed choices that echo in the steady rhythm of a healthy heart.

As we reflect on the plethora of recipes within these pages, it becomes apparent that eating for heart health is not about deprivation but about abundance. Abundance in colors, textures, and flavors that not only delight our senses but also contribute to the longevity and well-being of our most vital organ.

The vibrant array of fruits, vegetables, whole grains, and lean proteins serves as a reminder that a heart-healthy diet is diverse, exciting, and endlessly customizable to suit our individual tastes and preferences.

Moreover, this cookbook is not just a compilation of recipes; it is a manifesto for a lifestyle that prioritizes health without compromising on the joy of eating. It encourages us to be mindful of our food choices, to savor each bite, and to relish the connection between what we put on our plates and the vitality we feel within.

Through the incorporation of heart-boosting ingredients and culinary techniques, we are not only nurturing our physical health but also cultivating a profound relationship with the food we consume.

In the spirit of this heart-healthy culinary expedition, let us carry the lessons learned from these pages into our daily lives. May we approach our meals with a newfound awareness, recognizing that every choice we make in the kitchen has the power to shape our cardiovascular destiny.

As we savor the delectable dishes curated for heart wellness, may we find inspiration to experiment, innovate, and tailor these recipes to our individual tastes, ensuring that the journey to a healthier heart is as delightful as the destination itself.

In essence, this cookbook is an invitation a call to embrace a lifestyle where every meal is an act of self-love, a declaration of commitment to a heart that beats strong and true.

Let this culinary collection be a guide on your ongoing journey toward heart health, reminding you that in the realm of nourishment, each recipe is a step toward a vibrant, thriving, and heart fulfilled life.

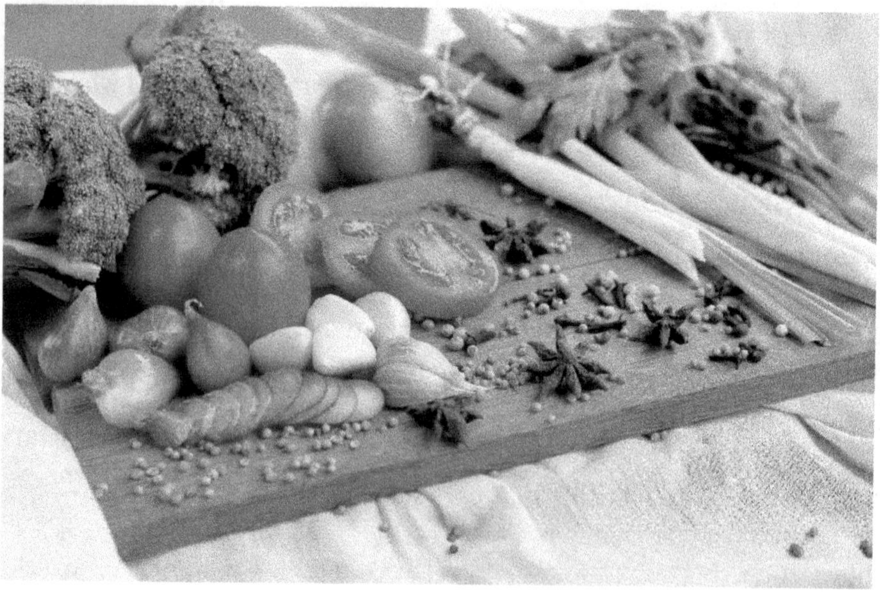

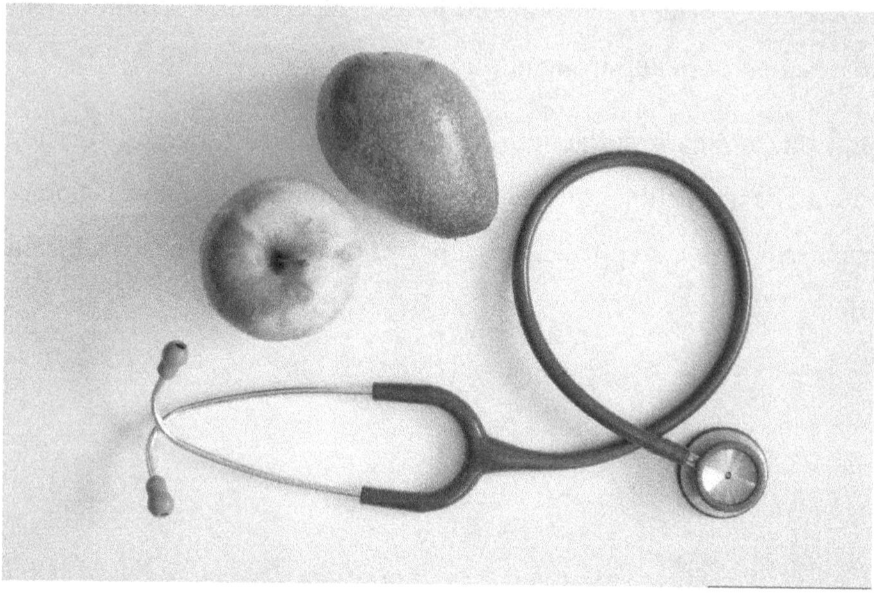

Weekly Meal Planner

	BREAKFAST	LUNCH	DINNER	SNACKS
MON				
TUE				
WED				
THU				
FRI				
SAT				
SUN				

Note:

Shopping list

Weekly Meal Planner

	BREAKFAST	LUNCH	DINNER	SNACKS
MON				
TUE				
WED				
THU				
FRI				
SAT				
SUN				

Note:

Shopping list

Weekly Meal Planner

	BREAKFAST	LUNCH	DINNER	SNACKS
MON				
TUE				
WED				
THU				
FRI				
SAT				
SUN				

Note:

Shopping list

Weekly Meal Planner

	BREAKFAST	LUNCH	DINNER	SNACKS
MON				
TUE				
WED				
THU				
FRI				
SAT				
SUN				

Note:

Shopping list

Weekly Meal Planner

	BREAKFAST	LUNCH	DINNER	SNACKS
MON				
TUE				
WED				
THU				
FRI				
SAT				
SUN				

Note:

Shopping list

Weekly Meal Planner

	BREAKFAST	LUNCH	DINNER	SNACKS
MON				
TUE				
WED				
THU				
FRI				
SAT				
SUN				

Note:

Shopping list